Novel Non-pharmacological Approaches to Heart Failure

Editors

VIJAY U. RAO
GEETHA BHAT

HEART FAILURE CLINICS

www.heartfailure.theclinics.com

Consulting Editor
EDUARDO BOSSONE

Founding Editor
JAGAT NARULA

January 2024 • Volume 20 • Number 1

ELSEVIER

1600 John F. Kennedy Boulevard • Suite 1800 • Philadelphia, Pennsylvania, 19103-2899

http://www.theclinics.com

HEART FAILURE CLINICS Volume 20, Number 1
January 2024 ISSN 1551-7136, ISBN-13: 978-0-443-18328-7

Editor: Joanna Gascoine
Developmental Editor: Nitesh Barthwal

Heart Failure Clinics (ISSN 1551-7136) is published quarterly by Elsevier Inc., 360 Park Avenue South, New York, NY 10010-1710. Months of publication are January, April, July, and October. Business and editorial offices: 1600 John F. Kennedy Boulevard, Suite 1800, Philadelphia, PA 19103-2899. Periodicals postage paid at New York, NY, and additional mailing offices. Subscription prices are USD 297.00 per year for US individuals, USD 100.00 per year for US students and residents, USD 324.00 per year for Canadian individuals, USD 341.00 per year for international individuals, and USD 100.00 per year for Canadian and foreign students/residents. For institutional access pricing please contact Customer Service via the contact information below. To receive student and resident rate, orders must be accompanied by name of affiliated institution, date of term, and the *signature* of program/residency coordinator on institution letterhead. Orders will be billed at individual rate until proof of status is received. Foreign air speed delivery is included in all *Clinics* subscription prices. All prices are subject to change without notice. **POSTMASTER:** Send address changes to *Heart Failure Clinics*, Elsevier Health Sciences Division, Subscription Customer Service, 3251 Riverport Lane, Maryland Heights, MO 63043. **Customer Service: 1-800-654-2452 (US and Canada). From outside of the US and Canada, call 314-447-8871. Fax: 314-447-8029. For print support, E-mail: JournalsCustomerService-usa@elsevier.com. For online support, E-mail: JournalsOnlineSupport-usa@elsevier.com.**

Reprints. For copies of 100 or more of articles in this publication, please contact the Commercial Reprints Department, Elsevier Inc., 360 Park Avenue South, New York, NY 10010-1710. Tel.: 212-633-3874; Fax: 212-633-3820; E-mail: reprints@elsevier.com.

Heart Failure Clinics is covered in *MEDLINE/PubMed (Index Medicus)*.

Contributors

CONSULTING EDITOR

EDUARDO BOSSONE, MD, PhD, FCCP, FESC, FACC
Consulting Editor, *Heart Failure Clinics*, Director of Cardiology, Cardarelli Hospital, Department of Public Health, Department of Translational Medical Sciences, University of Naples "Federico II," Naples, Italy

EDITORS

VIJAY U. RAO, MD, PhD, FACC, FASE, FHFSA, FICOS
Director, Heart Failure, CardioOncology, Anticoagulation, Franciscan Health, Indianapolis, Indiana, USA

GEETHA BHAT, PhD, MD, FACC, FAST, FHFSA
Program Director, Cardiac Transplantation, The Christ Hospital, Cincinnati, Ohio, USA

EDUARDO BOSSONE, MD, PhD, FCCP, FESC, FACC
Consulting Editor, *Heart Failure Clinics*, Director of Cardiology, Cardarelli Hospital, Department of Public Health, Department of Translational Medical Sciences, University of Naples "Federico II," Naples, Italy

AUTHORS

SATYANARAYANA ACHANTA, DVM, PhD, DABT
Assistant Professor, Department of Anesthesiology, Duke University School of Medicine, Durham, North Carolina, USA

ASIM S. AHMED, DO, FACC, FHRS
Cardiac Electrophysiologist, Director of Atrial Fibrillation Clinic, Department of Cardiac Electrophysiology, Ascension Sacred Heart Cardiology, Pensacola, Florida, USA

CATALIN F. BAICU, PhD
Associate Professor, Division of Cardiology, Department of Medicine, Medical University of South Carolina, The Ralph H. Johnson Department of Veterans Affairs Health Care System, Charleston, South Carolina, USA

CLAUDIA BARATTO, MD
Cardiologist, Division of Cardiology, Dyspnea and Pulmonary Hypertension Clinic, Ospedale San Luca IRCCS Istituto Auxologico Italiano, Milano, Italy

RONALD D. BASS, BA
School of Medicine, Georgetown University, NorthWest, Washington, DC, USA

JAN BIEGUS, MD
Assistant Professor, Institute of Heart Diseases, Wroclaw Medical University, Poland

ADAM BLAND, MBBS
Conjoint Associate Lecturer, Department of Cardiology, Gosford Hospital - Central Coast LHD, The University of Newcastle - Central Coast Clinical School, Gosford, New South Wales, Australia

SERGIO CARAVITA, MD, PhD
Cardiologist, Division of Cardiology, Dyspnea
and Pulmonary Hypertension Clinic, Ospedale
San Luca IRCCS Istituto Auxologico Italiano,
Milano, Italy; Department of Management,
Information and Production Engineering,
University of Bergamo, Dalmine, Province of
Bergamo, Italy

EUNICE CHUAH, MBBS
Department of Cardiology, Gosford Hospital -
Central Coast LHD, The University of
Newcastle - Central Coast Clinical School,
Gosford, New South Wales, Australia

RAFAEL DE LA ESPRIELLA, MD
Cardiologist, Cardiology Department, Hospital
Clínico Universitario de Valencia, Fundación de
Investigación INCLIVA, Valencia, Spain

THOMAS J. FORD, MBChB (Hons), PhD
Department of Cardiology, Gosford Hospital -
Central Coast LHD, The University of
Newcastle - Central Coast Clinical School,
Gosford, New South Wales, Australia;
University of Glasgow, ICAMS, Glasgow,
United Kingdom

MARAT FUDIM, MD, MHS
Cardiologist, Division of Cardiology,
Department of Medicine, Duke University, Duke
Clinical Research Institute, Durham, North
Carolina, USA

HECTOR M. GARCIA-GARCIA, MD, PhD
Professor, Interventional Cardiology, MedStar
Washington Hospital Center, Washington, DC,
USA

KASHVI GUPTA, MD, MPH
Saint Luke's Mid America Heart Institute,
University of Missouri-Kansas City, Kansas
City, Missouri, USA

GREGORY R. JACKSON, MD
Assistant Professor of Medicine, Medical
University of South Carolina, Director of Heart
Failure Programs, Ralph H. Johnson Veterans
Affairs Medical Center, Charleston, South
Carolina, USA

OMAR JAWAID, MD
Cardiologist, St. Vincents' Ascension,
Indianapolis, Indiana, USA

RAMI KAHWASH, MD
Professor in Internal Medicine, Division of
Cardiovascular Medicine, The Ohio State
University Wexner Medical Center, Columbus,
Ohio, USA

MUHAMMAD SHAHZEB KHAN, MBBS
Division of Cardiology, Department of
Medicine, Duke University, Durham, North
Carolina, USA

ANNE KROMAN, DO, PhD
Cardiologist, Division of Cardiology,
Department of Medicine, Medical University of
South Carolina, The Ralph H. Johnson
Department of Veterans Affairs Health Care
System, Charleston, South Carolina, USA

IOANNIS MASTORIS, MD
Cardiologist, Cardiology Division, Department
of Medicine, Massachusetts General Hospital,
Boston, Massachusetts, USA

WILLIAM MEERE, MBBS
Department of Cardiology, Gosford Hospital -
Central Coast LHD, The University of
Newcastle - Central Coast Clinical School,
Gosford, New South Wales, Australia

JULIO NÚÑEZ, MD
Cardiology Department, Hospital Clínico
Universitario de Valencia, Fundación de
Investigación INCLIVA, Department of
Medicine, University of Valencia, Valencia,
Spain; CIBER Cardiovascular, Madrid, Spain

ANOUSHEH AWAIS PARACHA, MBBS
Department of Medicine, Dow University of
Health Sciences, Karachi, Pakistan

PARIN J. PATEL, MD, FACC, FHRS
Cardiac Electrophysiologist, Director
Electrophysiology Laboratory, Department of
Cardiac Electrophysiology, Ascension St.
Vincent Heart Center, Indianapolis, Indiana,
USA

JOSEPH PHILLIPS, BS, MS
University of Iowa Hospitals and Clinics, Iowa
City, Iowa, USA

ASHWIN RAVICHANDRAN, MD
Cardiology Specialist, St. Vincents' Ascension,
Indianapolis, Indiana, USA

VINAY KUMAR REDDY VASANTHU, MBBS
Clinical Research Scholar, Department of
Anesthesiology, Duke University School of
Medicine, Durham, North Carolina, USA

KARL-PHILIPP ROMMEL, MD
Cardiologist, Department of Cardiology, Heart
Center at University of Leipzig, Leipzig Heart
Institute, Leipzig, Germany; Cardiovacular
Research Foundation, New York, New York, USA

JEAN M. RUDDY, MD
Vascular Surgery Specialist, Division of
Vascular Surgery, Department of Surgery,
Medical University of South Carolina, The
Ralph H. Johnson Department of Veterans
Affairs Health Care System, Charleston, South
Carolina, USA

HUSAM M. SALAH, MD
Cardiologist, Department of Internal Medicine,
University of Arkansas for Medical Sciences,
Little Rock, Arkansas, USA

CHRISTOPHER SALERNO, MD
Cardiac Surgeon, University of Chicago
Medical Center, Chicago, Illinois, USA

CARLOS G. SANTOS-GALLEGO, MD
Instructor, Cardiology Department, Mount Sinai
Hospital, Cardiovascular Institute, Icahn School
of Medicine at Mount Sinai, New York, New York,
USA

JORGE SANZ SÁNCHEZ, MD, PhD
Interventional Cardiologist, Hospital
Universitari I Politecnic La Fe, Valencia, Spain;
Centro de Investigación Biomedica en Red
(CIBERCV), Madrid, Spain

ANDREW J. SAUER, MD
Associate Professor, Saint Luke's Mid America
Heart Institute, University of Missouri-Kansas
City, Kansas City, Missouri, USA

SALVATORE SAVONA, MD
Cardiologist, Division of Cardiovascular
Medicine, The Ohio State University Wexner
Medical Center, Columbus, Ohio, USA

ABHINAV SINGH, MD, MPH
Medical Director, Indiana Sleep Center, Clinical
Assistant Professor, Marian University College
of Osteopathic Medicine, Greenwood, Indiana,
USA

PRITI SHAH, MSC
Infraredx, A Nipro Company, Bedford,
Massachusetts, USA

STEPHEN SUM, PhD
Infraredx, A Nipro Company, Bedford,
Massachusetts, USA

RON WAKSMAN, MD
Associate Director, Interventional Cardiology,
MedStar Washington Hospital Center,
Washington, DC, USA

ALEXANDER L. WALLNER, MD
Division of Cardiovascular Medicine, The Ohio
State University Wexner Medical Center,
Columbus, Ohio, USA

DMITRY M. YARANOV, MD
Cardiologist, Baptist Heart Institute, Baptist
Memorial Hospital, Baptist Memorial
Healthcare, Memphis, Tennessee, USA

MICHAEL R. ZILE, MD
Director of Cardiology, Division of Cardiology,
Department of Medicine, Medical University of
South Carolina, The Ralph H. Johnson
Department of Veterans Affairs Health Care
System, Charleston, South Carolina, USA

Contents

Targeted Therapies for Microvascular Disease

Adam Bland, Eunice Chuah, William Meere, and Thomas J. Ford

Coronary microvascular dysfunction (CMD) is a common cause of ischemia but no obstructive coronary artery disease that results in an inability of the coronary microvasculature to meet myocardial oxygen demand. CMD is challenging to diagnose and manage due to a lack of mechanistic research and targeted therapy. Recent evidence suggests we can improved patient outcomes by stratifying antianginal therapies according to the diagnosis revealed by invasive assessment of the coronary microcirculation. This review article appraises the evidence for management of CMD, which includes treatment of cardiovascular risk, antianginal therapy and therapy for atherosclerosis.

The Ability of Near-Infrared Spectroscopy to Identify Vulnerable Patients and Plaques: A Systematic Review and Meta-Analysis

Ronald D. Bass, Joseph Phillips, Jorge Sanz Sánchez, Priti Shah, Stephen Sum, Ron Waksman, and Hector M. Garcia-Garcia

Previous studies have analyzed the efficacy of near-infrared spectroscopy-derived lipid core burden index (LCBI) in quantifying and identifying high-risk plaques and patients at increased risk of future major adverse cardiac outcomes/major adverse cardiovascular and cerebrovascular events. A $maxLCBI_{4mm}$ of 400 or greater seems to be an effective threshold for classifying at-risk plaques. This meta-analysis provides a more precise odds ratio with a narrow standard deviation that can be used to guide future studies.

HEART FAILURE CLINICS

SERIES OF RELATED INTEREST

Cardiology Clinics
http://www.cardiology.theclinics.com/
Cardiac Electrophysiology Clinics
https://www.cardiacep.theclinics.com/
Interventional Cardiology Clinics
https://www.interventional.theclinics.com/

THE CLINICS ARE AVAILABLE ONLINE!
Access your subscription at:
www.theclinics.com

Preface

Interventional Approaches to Augment Pharmacotherapy in Heart Failure

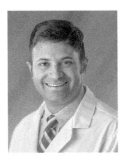

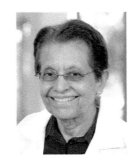

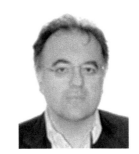

Vijay U. Rao, MD, PhD, FACC, FASE, FHFSA, FICOS

Geetha Bhat, PhD, MD, FACC, FAST, FHFSA

Eduardo Bossone, MD, PhD, FCCP, FESC, FACC

Editors

Heart Failure (HF) morbidity and mortality remain high, exacting an enormous toll on both patients and health care systems globally. Over the last decade, marked advances in our understanding of HF pathophysiology and phenotypes have led to novel pharmacologic options for patients with both HF with reduced ejection fraction and HF with preserved ejection fraction.[1,2] Many efforts are underway to improve uptake of guideline-directed medical therapy with the potential to meaningfully impact patient outcomes. Equally impressive, however, is the explosion of research into novel nonpharmacologic treatments for HF that are rapidly moving into the clinical arena. Given that many HF providers may not be aware of many of these new treatment options, herein, we provide a 2023 update.

In this issue of *Heart Failure Clinics*, you hear from Dr Gupta and colleagues about recent advances in remote monitoring devices, both noninvasive and invasive, and how they might be used to track actionable data to predict HF decompensation, guide diuretic management, and prevent hospital admissions. Atrial fibrillation often coexists with HF and has been shown to impact HF outcomes. Drs Patel and Ahmed provide an update on interventional approaches to maintaining sinus rhythm in HF patients (pulmonary vein isolation ablation) as well as when atrial-ventricular node

ablation followed by chronic resynchronization therapy would be indicated. Obstructive sleep apnea (OSA) is a key driver of both HF and atrial fibrillation. We are fortunate to hear from both an HF cardiologist (Dr Jackson) and a sleep medicine specialist (Dr Singh) on why diagnosing and treating OSA is critically important to our HF patients. They describe the different types of apnea (central and obstructive) as well as advances in devices currently being used to treat sleep apnea.

Next, Dr Salah and colleagues provide an update on the promise and pitfalls of interatrial shunt devices with a focus on reducing left atrial pressure that could impact left atrial remodeling and ultimately improve exercise tolerance in HF patients. This section is followed by Dr Khan and colleagues who describe how preload reduction strategies that reduce inflow into the heart or increase splanchnic vascular blood pooling ultimately reduce intracardiac filling pressures and may thus present a unique opportunity to impact HF patients.

These sections are followed by a review of baroreflex activation therapy by Dr Ruddy and colleagues. They describe how a surgically placed extravascular lead can modulate autonomic nervous system imbalance to improve exercise capacity, quality of life, and functional class in HF patients. This is followed by a review of cardiac

Heart Failure Clin 20 (2024) xi–xii
https://doi.org/10.1016/j.hfc.2023.07.001
1551-7136/24/© 2023 Published by Elsevier Inc.

heartfailure.theclinics.com

contractility modulation therapy by Dr Wallner and colleagues in which nonexcitatory electrical myocardial stimulation increases contractility and improves HF symptoms in patients with left ventricular ejection fraction between 25% and 45% who remain symptomatic despite optimal medical therapy.

Last, we hear from Dr Jawaid and colleagues on left ventricular assist device therapy (LVAD) both as destination therapy and as a bridge to heart transplantation. Advances in devices have begun to address many of the prior limitations of LVADs, such as thrombosis and stroke rates, need for reoperation, and gastrointestinal bleeding. Fully internalized devices may soon be on the horizon.

While HF outcomes remain a major challenge, as this issue illustrates, there has never been a better time for optimism given the creativity, ingenuity, and passion of the HF research and development space.

Vijay U. Rao, MD, PhD, FACC, FASE, FHFSA, FICOS
Heart Failure, CardioOncology, Anticoagulation
Franciscan Health
5330 East Stop 11 Road
Indianapolis, IN 46235, USA

Geetha Bhat, PhD, MD, FACC, FAST, FHFSA
Cardiac Transplantation
The Christ Hospital
2139 Auburn Avenue
Cincinnati, OH 45219, USA

Eduardo Bossone, MD, PhD, FCCP, FESC, FACC
Department of Public Health
Department of Translational Medical Sciences
University of Naples "Federico II"
Ed. 18, I piano, Via Sergio Pansini 5, Naples
80131, Italy

E-mail addresses:
veej7474@hotmail.com (V.U. Rao)
geethabhat72@gmail.com (G. Bhat)
eduardo.bossone@unina.it (E. Bossone)

REFERENCES

1. Sharma A, Verma S, Bhatt DL, et al. Optimizing foundational therapies in patients with HFrEF: how do we translate these findings into clinical care? JACC Basic Transl Sci 2022;7(5):504–17.
2. Bhatt AS, Abraham WT, Lindenfeld J, et al. Treatment of HF in an era of multiple therapies: statement from the HF Collaboratory. JACC Heart Fail 2021;9(1):1–12.

Remote Monitoring Devices and Heart Failure

Kashvi Gupta, MD, MPH[a], Ioannis Mastoris, MD[b], Andrew J. Sauer, MD[a],*

KEYWORDS

- Remote monitoring • Heart failure • Pulmonary artery pressure monitoring
- Intrathoracic impedance

KEY POINTS

- Remote patient monitoring (RPM) devices in heart failure (HF) have evolved in the last 2 decades from vital sign monitoring devices to more sophisticated invasive and noninvasive devices to identify and intervene on patients before a worsening HF event.
- Patient and device selection, along with a structured protocol for intervening on values above a predefined threshold for physiological parameters being measured, are key to success with RPM.
- Reorganizing HF clinics and having dedicated telemonitoring device teams are needed for improving clinic workflows.

INTRODUCTION

Remote patient monitoring (RPM) involves intervening in a patient's health status through non–face-to-face interaction utilizing transmission of physiological data or patient-reported symptoms via telemedicine platforms for ongoing management of chronic conditions.[1] Using RPM, physiological data can be continuously captured using wearable or implantable devices. These data generated from RPM devices are then transferred to the health-care provider via a wireless connection that triggers a targeted follow-up based on deviations from preset thresholds. Telemonitoring is beneficial for engaging patients in their medical management, symptom monitoring, intensification or optimization of guideline-directed medical therapy (GDMT), and reduction of risk for hospitalization before worsening of symptoms in chronic medical conditions such as heart failure (HF).[2,3]

HF affects more than 6 million people in the United States (~1.8% of the US population using the 2020 Census) with a projected increase to more than 8 million by 2030.[4,5] Racial and gender differences in the incidence and prevalence of HF have been previously shown; Blacks and women with HF experience worse health outcomes as compared with Whites and men, respectively.[6] The cost associated with HF was estimated around US$30.7 billion in 2012, mostly attributed to direct medical costs related to hospitalizations. The former is expected to increase to US$69.8 billion (an increase of 127%) by 2030 baring modifications to the HF care paradigm.[7,8] These morbidity, mortality, and economic burdens are attributed principally to HF readmissions, a vulnerable period following an index HF hospitalization. In 2017, the 30-day and 90-day readmission rates were 18% and 31%, respectively. These have not only significantly increased since 2010 but also expected to increase with an aging population and increased prevalence of HF.[9] Accordingly, developing strategies to reduce readmissions and improve the health outcomes of patients with HF is a national priority.

The initial large-scale randomized clinical trials evaluating RPM in HF took place at a time when the Centers for Medicare and Medicaid Services

a Saint Luke's Mid America Heart Institute, University of Missouri-Kansas City, Kansas City, MO, USA;
b Cardiology Division, Department of Medicine, Massachusetts General Hospital, Boston, MA, USA
* Corresponding author. 4401 Wornall Road, Kansas City, MO 64111.
E-mail address: asauer@saint-lukes.org

Heart Failure Clin 20 (2024) 1–13
https://doi.org/10.1016/j.hfc.2023.05.002

heartfailure.theclinics.com

(CMS), in 2004, implemented pilot projects that used monitoring technologies (such as vital signs, symptomatic information, and health self-assessment) to enable remote guidance of patients with chronic health conditions.[10] In 2009, CMS publicly reported hospital rates of HF mortality and readmissions as part of its quality initiative to evaluate hospital-level performance across the country.[11] In 2010, the Patient Protection and Affordable Care Act[12] was signed into law, establishing financial incentives for hospitals nationwide to reduce HF-related readmission rates. The early trials evaluating RPM have thus focused on improving the transition of care from inpatient to outpatient, utilizing existing technologies to reduce readmission and mortality rates. During the last 2 decades, the use of devices in RPM in HF has evolved based on accumulated evidence and technological advancements, from vital signs monitoring to more complex interventions using implantable devices to measure cardiac filling pressures.

Today, remote monitoring devices in HF can be broadly classified into noninvasive or wearable devices and invasive or implantable devices. Further, devices can be classified based on the parameters of interest, such as vital signs, hemodynamics, lung congestion biomarkers, and arrhythmia burden. The choice of device(s) used to monitor a patient can be system based, depending on a health system intervention as studied in clinical trials, or individualized for the patient depending on HF cause, stage, medical therapy, access, and affordability.

DISCUSSION
Noninvasive Remote Patient Monitoring Devices

The most basic form of RPM, having undergone investigation in patients with HF, is the monitoring of vital signs using electronic weighing scales, blood pressure cuffs, heart rate monitors, electrocardiograms (ECGs), and pulse oximeters. Randomized clinical trials that implemented telemonitoring using electronic equipment that measured daily blood pressure, heart rate, ECGs, symptoms, and body weight have shown the feasibility of such interventions. However, for the most part, they have failed to show efficacy in reducing readmissions or all-cause mortality compared with usual care.[13–20] It is worth noting that these trials were conducted in a different era of telemonitoring, and with complex interventions, efficacy depends on the context in which the intervention is applied. For example, the early trials were heterogenous in their approaches to patient selection, deployed a variety of clinical workflows,

and the use of data acquired through telemonitoring to modify HF treatment to affect outcome was also variable. After these trials were conducted, there have been foundational changes in the management of HF such as device technologies have evolved, our ability to integrate multiple data sources into the electronic medical record and other platforms have advanced, and our understanding of the different phenotypes of HF and their management strategies have been updated.[21]

The timeline of clinical trials that evaluated vital sign monitoring to reduce all-cause mortality and HF-related events is depicted in **Fig. 1**. The Weight Monitoring in Heart Failure (WHARF) trial[13] in 1998 was the first multicenter clinical trial to study a technology-based remote monitoring strategy for patients with HF using patient-reported symptoms and weight. Subsequent clinical trials have built on earlier interventions to address limitations and improve the delivery of telemonitoring with current technologies. For example, we can compare and contrast the Telemedical Interventional Monitoring in Heart Failure (TIM-HF) trial[19] and the TIM-HF II trial.[22] The trials differed in patient selection, follow-up duration, and telemonitoring devices. Both studies included patients with New York Heart Association (NYHA) functional classes II or III. Although the TIM-HF trial further included patients with left ventricular ejection fraction (LVEF) of 35% or lesser and a minimum of one HF admission within 24 months of randomization or those with an LVEF of 25% or lesser without a mandatory recent hospitalization, the TIM-HF II trial included those with EF of 45% or lesser or LVEF greater than 45% and diuretic use. Specifically, TIM-HF II excluded patients with major depression from the trial. Those with such mental health conditions tended to have higher readmission rates in a subgroup analysis of TIM-HF. Regarding the follow-up duration, while TIM-HF utilized a fixed stop date and had a median follow-up of 26 months, TIM-HF II had a follow-up of 12 months for participants. Finally, in TIM-HF, patients utilized a landline to contact the emergency response system, while in the TIM-HF II trial, all patients received a mobile phone. The TIM-HF II trial concluded that a structured telemonitoring plan reduces hospitalization and all-cause mortality in a carefully selected HF population. In aggregate, although there has been a paucity of evidence to support monitoring of patient vitals to improve HF clinical outcomes (specifically readmissions and mortality), there remains an opportunity for further investigation with emphasis on patient selection, newer technologies, and structured interventions that can ensure higher adherence rates to the intervention.

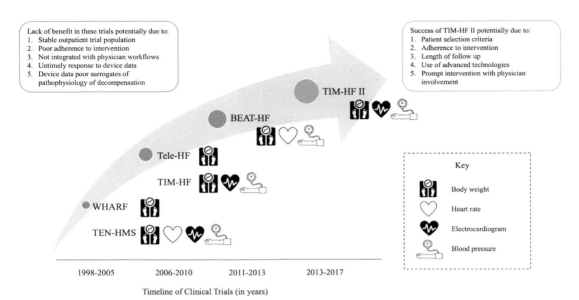

Lack of benefit in these trials potentially due to:
1. Stable outpatient trial population
2. Poor adherence to intervention
3. Not integrated with physician workflows
4. Untimely response to device data
5. Device data poor surrogates of pathophysiology of decompensation

Success of TIM-HF II potentially due to:
1. Patient selection criteria
2. Adherence to intervention
3. Length of follow up
4. Use of advanced technologies
5. Prompt intervention with physician involvement

TIM-HF II
BEAT-HF
Tele-HF
TIM-HF
WHARF
TEN-HMS

Key

Body weight

Heart rate

Electrocardiogram

Blood pressure

1998-2005   2006-2010   2011-2013   2013-2017

Timeline of Clinical Trials (in years)

Fig. 1. Clinical trials evaluating noninvasive telemonitoring. List of clinical trials referenced in the figure. BEAT-HF, The Better Effectiveness After Transition–Heart Failure20; Tele-HF, Telemonitoring to Improve Heart Failure Outcomes 15; TEN-HMS, The Trans-European Network-Home-Care Management System 26; TIM-HF, Telemedical Interventional Monitoring in Heart Failure 19; TIM-HF II, Telemedical Interventional Monitoring in Heart Failure 2 22; WHARF, The Weight Monitoring in Heart Failure trial 13.

Body weight—an unreliable surrogate of cardiac filling pressures

The general premise for remote monitoring of vitals is to reduce HF-related hospitalizations that result from acute HF decompensation. In effect, the goal is to capture physiological data for early detection of clinical deterioration that can be corrected with interventions provided by physicians remotely to the patient.[23] However, the measurement of body weight as a surrogate of volume status or left ventricular filling pressure to guide titration of diuretics at home has been debated.[24–26] Overall, weight gain alone is neither a sensitive nor a specific marker, even when coupled with other vitals, to reduce HF-related hospitalizations. In comparison, invasive remote monitoring devices offer a greater insight into a patient's volume status at an earlier stage.[27]

Invasive Remote Patient Monitoring Devices

Invasive RPM uses implantable devices that measure parameters such as hemodynamics, lung congestion, and arrhythmia burden. These devices rely on the principle of subclinical detection of increased cardiac filling pressures, as shown in **Fig. 2**. Modern cardiac implantable electronic devices (CIEDs) that include cardiac resynchronization therapy (CRT) or implantable cardioverter defibrillator (ICD) have been upgraded with expanded monitoring capabilities of physiologic

parameters such as thoracic impedance, arrhythmia burden, heart rate variability, and physical activity levels. These CIEDs that facilitate continuous monitoring of physiological data provide an opportunity for telemonitoring in HF. We discuss below devices used for hemodynamic monitoring (right ventricle pressure monitoring, left atrial (LA) pressure monitoring, and pulmonary artery [PA] pressure monitoring) and CIEDs (thoracic impedance monitoring, other physiologic parameters, and heart rhythms).

Right ventricle pressure monitoring

The Chronicle Offers Management to Patients with Advanced Signs and Symptoms of Heart Failure Study (COMPASS-HF)[28] was a landmark study that evaluated the use of a hemodynamic monitoring system, the Chronicle, to determine a patient's cardiac pressure status remotely and intervene accordingly to prevent HF-related events. Details about the device are included in **Table 1**. The trial enrolled patients (regardless of EF) with functional status NYHA III or IV that were noninotrope dependent. In the intervention arm (n = 134/274), data collected from the device was uploaded to a web platform and reviewed at least once a week by clinicians. Although the trial met its safety endpoint, it did not meet the primary efficacy endpoint during a 6-month follow-up period. The lessons learned from the trial include first, right-sided pressures may not have been

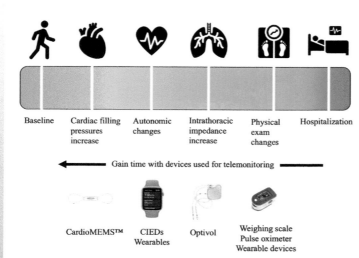

Fig. 2. Remote hemodynamic monitoring from chronic compensated to acute decompensated HF and example of devices used across the spectrum for telemonitoring Abbreviations: CIEDS, cardiac implantable electronic devices.

accurately measured to provide the required information for averting an HF hospitalization; second, there was a gradual increase in mean PA pressure that correlated with events; and third, there could be a gap between increasing cardiac filling pressures and physicians recognizing these patterns to intervene with adjustment of medications before HF decompensation occurs.[29]

Left atrial pressure monitoring

Monitoring the LA pressure can provide insight into the hemodynamics of the left side of the heart. These can be calculated using transthoracic echocardiograms (TTEs) or implantable devices. Because TTEs are not practical to obtain in an RPM environment, implantable devices that measure LA pressure can assist in telemonitoring. The risks associated with these devices include thromboembolism, bleeding, and catheter retention at the time of removal. Refer to **Table 1** for a description of these devices and associated clinical trials.

The Hemodynamically Guided Home Self-Therapy in Severe Heart Failure Patients (HOMEO-STASIS) trial[30] evaluated continuous LA pressure monitoring using the HeartPOD device to allow earlier identification of impending HF decompensation that can guide adjustment of diuretics to reduce HF-related events. Implantation of the device (n = 40) was shown to be feasible and safe.[30,31] Further, the trial showed improved survival in the intervention arm at 3 years, with a significantly decreased frequency of HF-related events within the first 3 months (HR: 0.16; 95% CI: 0.04–0.68).[30]

The Left Atrial Pressure Monitoring to Optimize Heart Failure Therapy Study (LAPTOP-HF)[32,33] studied the safety and efficacy of a LAP monitoring

system in measuring LA pressure to optimize medical therapy and prevent HF decompensation in patients with functional status NYHA III regardless of EF. LAPTOP-HF enrolled 486 of the planned 730 patients because the study was terminated early due to perceived excess device-related complications. All participants that were registered were followed for a period of 12 months. The study found that implanting the LAP monitoring system was safe and effective in reducing HF-related hospitalizations (P = .005).

The V-LAP Left Atrium Monitoring systEm for Patients With Chronic sysTOlic & Diastolic Congestive heart Failure (VECTOR-HF) trial[34] studied the safety and efficacy of the V-LAP system in patients with NYHA III HF (irrespective of EF) and hospitalization for HF within 12 months or elevated natriuretic peptide. The trial enrolled 24 patients in whom the LA pressure was reported to be accurate and was concordant with the wedge pressure (correlation coefficient = 0.85) at 3 months. Further, in a patient who completed the 6-month follow-up, there was an improvement in the NYHA functional status. A unique feature of the V-LAP system is that patients can monitor their LA pressure data on their mobile applications to adjust their diuretic doses when the pressure is out of normal range. This allows patients to be actively involved in their HF management. They are advised to contact their health-care provider for high or low readings.

Pulmonary artery pressure monitoring

Elevated PA diastolic pressure of 15 mm Hg or greater, which reflects increased LA pressure, is a marker of hemodynamic congestion. The CardioMEMS Heart Sensor Allows Monitoring of Pressure to Improve Outcomes in NYHA Class III

Table 1
Description of devices and associated trials used for invasive hemodynamic monitoring

Device	Device Description	Monitoring Parameters	Clinical Trial, Year	Key Findings
Chronicle[26]	• RV hemodynamic monitoring system • A transvenous lead that is positioned in the RVOT or septum and has a sensor incorporated at its tip • Device is positioned subcutaneously in the pectoral muscle • An external pressure reference device is also carried by the patient • A home monitor interrogates the device via a radiofrequency wand and transmits the data through a telephone line to a secure server	• Heart rate, body temperature, physical activity • RV systolic and diastolic pressure • Using an algorithm, it calculates the ePAD using RV pressures	COMPASS-HF, 2003–2005	At 6 mo, patients in the intervention arm had a 21% lower incidence of the composite primary endpoint of HF related hospitalization, ER visits, or urgent care visits; however, this finding did not meet statistical significance
HeartPOD[28,29]	• LA hemodynamic monitoring system • An implantable sensor lead positioned in the atrial septum and oriented to the LA • Subcutaneous antenna coil that is placed in a pocket in the lower abdomen	• Heart rate, body temperature, intracardiac ECG • LA pressure calculated by subtracting absolute pressure from atmospheric pressure measured using a patient advisory module	HOMEOSTASIS, 2005–2007	At 3 y, there was improved LA pressure control, reduced HF symptoms, more optimal titration of diuretics, and reduction in HF-related clinical events

(continued on next page)

Table 1
(continued)

Device	Device Description	Monitoring Parameters	Clinical Trial, Year	Key Findings
LAP Monitoring System [32,33]	• LA hemodynamic monitoring system • An implantable sensor lead (same as HeartPOD) positioned in the atrial septum and oriented to the LA • The lead is coupled to an implanted communications module that transfers collected data to an external radiofrequency reader. The communications module is implanted in the pectoral muscle • If the implanting physician additionally decided on CRT and opted to place a single device, the LAP combination system was used. This consisted of a Promote CRT-D LAP pulse generator that accommodated 3 market-approved pacing/defibrillating leads and the implantable sensor lead	• Heart rate, body temperature, intracardiac ECG • LA pressure waveform	LAPTOP-HF, 2010–2015	At 12 mo, LA pressure monitoring using the LAP Monitoring system was safe and associated with 41% reduction in HF-related hospitalizations. Enrollment was stopped early due to a perceived excess of procedure-related complications
V-LAP [34]	• LA hemodynamic monitoring system • The sensory implant is placed in the LA septum, and it transmits LA pressure to an external unit • The external unit is worn by the patient on a belt across the torso • The external unit powers the implant and collects data via radiofrequency communication	• LA pressure waveform	VECTOR-HF, 2019–2020	Data obtained from the sensor correlated with LA pressure and had good concordance with the wedge pressure. In patients who completed the 6-mo follow-up, there was improvement in the NYHA functional class

Device	Description	Parameters	Trials	Outcomes
	• Data from the external unit is then transferred to the cloud and made available in the patient's mobile application			
CardioMEMS HF System [35,37]	• PA hemodynamic monitoring system • An implantable sensor coil and pressure-sensitive capacitor placed into a distal PA branch • PA pressure is recorded when the patient lies in a supine position • Readings are immediately transmitted to a secure internet database	• Heart rate • PA systolic, diastolic, and mean pressures	CHAMPION, 2007–2009 GUIDE-HF, 2018–2019	CHAMPION: At 6 mo, patients in the intervention arm had a 37% reduction in HF-related hospitalizations GUIDE-HF: At 12 mo, lower HF-related hospitalization and urgent HF visits in the intervention arm as compared with placebo, that was not statically significant
Cordella HF System and Cordella Pulmonary Artery Pressure Sensor [40,41]	• Comprehensive digital HF management system that records vital signs and a PA hemodynamic monitoring system • The Cordella PA pressure sensor is implanted in the right PA • Daily PA pressure is recorded by the patient, while seated, holding the wireless hand-held sensor reading device against the right pectoral region for 20 s • Vital signs are recorded by the Cordella HF system • Data are compiled and transmitted to a patient management portal	• Blood pressure, heart rate, body weight, oxygen saturation • KCCQ score • PA systolic, diastolic, and mean pressures	SIRONA, 2017–2019 SIRONA 2, 2019–2021	The Cordella PA pressure device has high adherence rate, equivocal readings to right heart catheterization, and implanting the device is safe and feasible

Abbreviations: CRT, cardiac resynchronization therapy; ePAD, estimated pulmonary arterial diastolic pressure; ER, emergency room; HF, heart failure; KCCQ, Kansas city cardiomyopathy questionnaire; LA, left atrium; PA, pulmonary artery; RV, right ventricle; RVOT right ventricle outflow tract.
Data from Refs.[28,30–35,37,40,41]

Heart Failure Patients (CHAMPION) trial[35] hypothesized that in patients with recent HF-related hospitalization, monitoring of PA pressure would reduce rehospitalization for HF. In 6 months, the trial demonstrated a 39% reduction in HF-related hospitalization in the CardioMEMS arm compared with usual care. During an additional mean follow-up of 13 months where physicians had open access to data from the control group, HF-related hospitalizations decreased by 48% (HR 0.52, 95% CI 0.40–0.69) compared with rates during the randomized control trial.[36] The CHAMPION trial was the first positive randomized control trial that confirmed implanting the hemodynamic monitoring system, CardioMEMS, was safe, and incorporating its data into clinical practice improved outcomes for patients with HF (with reduced and preserved EF) and NYHA class III.[35–37]

To study the benefit of CardioMEMS in patients with HF and NYHA class II-IV, the hemodynamic-GUIDEed management of Heart Failure (GUIDE-HF) trial[38] was undertaken from March 2018 to December 2019, and the follow-up of the trial was completed in January 2021. The trial was affected by the coronavirus disease-2019 (COVID-19) pandemic. At 12 months, the study found lower events of HF-related hospitalizations or urgent HF visits in patients in the CardioMEMS arm compared with usual care. However, the finding did not meet statistical significance. However, in a pre-COVID-19 substudy analysis, the pre-COVID-19 era, there was a significant reduction in the primary outcome driven by lower HF-related hospitalizations. Today, the CardioMEMS is the only FDA-approved device for monitoring intracardiac filling pressures for patients with functional status of NYHA II or III and who have been hospitalized for HF in the earlier 12 months or have elevated natriuretic peptides.[39]

The SIRONA trial[40] was designed to test the safety and accuracy of the Cordella HF System and Cordella PA Pressure Sensor in patients with HF and NYHA III functional status. In 15 patients recruited to the trial between 2017 and 2019, it demonstrated accuracy in recording PA pressure, safety in implanting the devices, 99% adherence to the intervention, and improvements in the health status of patients with lowering of the PA pressure. The SIRONA 2 trial[41] conducted between 2019 and 2021 showed similar findings in a larger trial population (n = 70) of patients with HF with NYHA III functional status. The prospective, multicenter, open-label, single-arm clinical trial evaluating the safety and efficacy of the Cordella pulmonary artery sensor system in NYHA class III heart failure patients (PROACTIVE-HF) trial[42] is ongoing. It will provide further insights into the benefits of combining vital sign measurement with PA pressure monitoring for the management of patients with HF and NYHA III functional status. The study started enrolling participants in January 2020 and is expected to finish enrollment by March 2023, with follow-up completion in March 2026.[43] **Table 1** describes the Cordella HF system and sensors and CardioMEMS device.

Cardiac implantable electronic devices for telemonitoring

Worsening pulmonary congestion can be detected using intrathoracic impedance. Accumulating fluid in the intrathoracic space hinders the flow of electrical current while crossing the lung and decreases impedance (effective resistance of the circuit) because fluid offers better conductance. Studies have shown a good correlation between intrathoracic impedance monitoring and capillary wedge pressures in patients with HF decompensation.[44,45] For example, the Medtronic Impedance Diagnostics in Heart Failure study suggested intrathoracic impedance may represent a surrogate measure of pulmonary fluid status in hospitalized patients with HF.[44] Accordingly, CIEDs can also detect thoracic impedance that can assist clinicians with monitoring and intervening in lung congestion in HF.[46] Clinical trials that have utilized CIEDs for intrathoracic impedance monitoring are summarized below.

The Sensitivity of the InSync Sentry OptiVol feature for the prediction of Heart Failure trial[47] evaluated the OptiVol feature in select CRT-D and ICD devices in patients with a recent HF hospitalization requiring titration of inotropes, nitrates, or diuretics. The study found an intrathoracic impedance-based fluid index had low sensitivity of 20.7% at the start of the study that increased to only 42.1% at 6 months postimplant.[47] The Diagnostic Outcome Trial in Heart Failure trial studied intrathoracic impedance monitoring in patients with an LVEF of 35% or lesser at the time of implantation of an ICD alone or with CRT using the audible alerts for guiding interventions to reduce HF-related hospitalizations. The trial led to increased health-care utilization and downstream hospitalizations for HF. The use of alerts in impedance monitoring from CIEDs was also not found to be superior to routine care in the Optimization of Heart Failure trial[48] or the MOnitoring Resynchronization dEvices and CARdiac patiEnts (MORE-CARE) randomized controlled trial.[49] In contrast, the remote management of heart failure using implantable electronic devices trial[50] did not use alerts to trigger interaction with a health-care provider and instead utilized trends in hemodynamic parameters obtained from the CIEDs. Still, their study also failed to show a reduction in all-cause mortality or HF-related hospitalizations.

Why did these trials not show a benefit? Apart from factors related to the trial designs, the following should be considered: (1) daily impedance monitoring may not be a valuable marker of impending HF decompensation; (2) the thresholds used to alert patients and physicians (60 Ω-days) might not be optimal; (3) patient selection might have played a role; (4) a multidisciplinary team of HF specialists and electrophysiologists may not have been available at all sites; (5) data overload might have hampered interpretation and meaningful intervention; and (6) the time lag of data transmission and intervention by physicians based on their individual decision-making rather than a structured protocol could also have contributed to suboptimal management in some patients.

The use of a multisensory HF index and alert algorithm (HeartLogic) to risk stratify patients based on HF events and to identify those with a meaningfully higher risk on follow-up was studied in the Multisensor Chronic Evaluation in Ambulatory Heart Failure Patients trial.[51] The HeartLogic uses data gathered from multiple sensors embedded within the CRT-D that captures several pathophysiological parameters of HF, such as heart sounds, respiratory rate, tidal volume, intrathoracic impedance, heart rate, and physical activity. These yield a HeartLogic HF index that is calculated daily, and if a patient's value deviates from baseline, an alert is issued. The study found that the HeartLogic HF index score could identify those with a 10-fold higher risk of worsening HF-related events. When the score was combined with N-terminal pro-B-type natriuretic peptide, it identified those with worsening HF-related events by a 50-fold increase. These algorithms can be used to triage resources to those at higher risk of HF-related decompensation.[51] The application of the HeartLogic HF index and the alert algorithm was then studied in the phase one trial, Multiple cArdiac seNsors for mAnaGEment of Heart Failure (MANAGE-HF) study.[52] The study found it safe to implement the score, resulting in faster intensification of GDMT with subsequent reduction of the HeartLogic HF index.[52] The index and alert algorithm application in a larger clinical trial are ongoing.

Future Directions Involving Less-Invasive Monitoring and Areas for Improvement

RPM in HF has come a long way, from having patients monitor their body weight at home to having them monitor and self-manage their cardiac filling pressures using mobile phone-based applications. The future of RPM depends on creating an intuitive environment for physicians and patients to use, developing creative solutions for curating and integrating data silos, and aligning payment models.

Wearables
Consumer-grade wearables are electronic devices with sophisticated sensors, intricately linked software systems, and compact hardware designs worn on the body as an accessory or embedded into clothing to track an array of health metrics. Wearables can measure physical activity, heart rate, heart rate variability, heart rhythms, and blood pressure that can be used for risk stratification in patients with HF. However, there are limited studies to suggest the utility of wearables in the HF population because technological advancements in the wearable arena have far outpaced evidence-based medicine. Accordingly, although we have a vast supply of wearable data, we have sparse outcomes data for most wearables.[53,54]

Several challenges hinder the widespread use of wearables in clinical practice. These challenges include data accuracy, data security, limited clinical trial evidence for devices related to specific disease processes, costs to maintain the machine and supporting software platforms, and integration of data from devices into clinical workflows.[55] Future studies could assess the value of wearables in RPM in HF, from simple vital sign monitoring to understanding heart rate variability and recovery and identifying arrhythmias to risk stratify patients for CRT.

Clinical workflows
Outside of the clinical trial environment that has organized clinical workflows around their specific intervention, clinical workflows for RPM patients with HF in the day-to-day practice need improvement. Physicians using RPM devices have reorganized their clinic structure, including staffing, to incorporate telemonitoring into their routine. For example, HF clinics have a nurse or a team of nurses who perform several tasks, as illustrated in **Fig. 3**. After implantation, they assist with patient education regarding the device and the integration of data obtained from cloud servers linked to telemonitoring devices into the electronic medical record. The nurse is also trained to either flag values for review by physicians or intervene based on structured protocols. Future device algorithms can be optimized to involve health-care providers only when there is data that are action-oriented. Improving such clinical workflows will make RPM more attractive to health-care providers and patients.

Artificial intelligence
Artificial intelligence (AI) plays many roles in cardiovascular medicine, such as risk prediction,

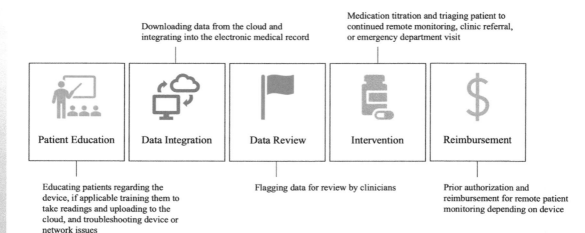

Fig. 3. HF clinic workflow for RPM device team.

triaging, diagnostics, and improving workflows. A primary application of good AI would be to sort actionable data from noise and enhance RPM interventions. The opportunities for the application of AI in the management of patients with HF in the telehealth environment are ongoing, and future studies can highlight the integration of AI algorithms into RPM interventions.[56]

Reassessing designs and endpoints of telemonitoring trials

An aspect of telemonitoring trials is to monitor changes in hemodynamics to predict HF decompensation and to intervene promptly to prevent it. Another element is also coaching patients to drive behavior change. For example, the Electronically Delivered Patient-Activation Tool for Intensification of Medications for Chronic Heart Failure with Reduced Ejection Fraction trial[57] studied the impact of engaging patients in optimizing their GDMT through review of electronically delivered 3-minute videos and checklists. The trial showed that their patient activation tool improved the intensification of GDMT.

Microrandomized trials can be used to study the needs and desires of individuals based on their responses to different personalizations and recommendations of an intervention.[58] Moreover, understanding the optimal dose of digital engagement to drive behavioral changes and maintain long-term adherence to digital interventions will require qualitative studies. These qualitative studies in the future can also shed light on data autonomy or the quantity and types of data a patient is comfortable self-managing.

Readmissions and mortality are essential health-care outcomes because they are expensive and often preventable adverse events following an index HF hospitalization. However, many factors influence HF-related readmissions, including patient-related ones (medical complexity, disability, affordability, and access) and community factors (neighborhood socioeconomic variables).[59] Evaluating the efficacy of RPM interventions solely based on a composite primary outcome of readmission and mortality rates reflects on hospital performances rather than the intervention itself. Further, these outcomes might only be evident during short follow-up periods. Overall, using all-cause-based outcomes sets a high bar for RPM interventions that can potentially reduce individual patient risk for the progression of HF and improve patient-reported health status outcomes.[60] Future studies must evaluate outcomes that are meaningful to the intervention and from the patient and provider perspective (such as GDMT titration) rather than a health system perspective (such as readmission rates) alone.

Reimbursements and health policy

There needs to be a better alignment of payment systems with the value RPM is bringing to the health system at different time points. If actionable care is aligned with reimbursements, there would be cost savings for the entire system. Increasingly, federal lawmakers are taking an interest in telehealth and are addressing these barriers.[1,61] During the COVID-19 pandemic, both the CMS and private insurance companies established telehealth payment models that were most recently extended for another 1 to 2 years.[62] Future research can inform the government on the impact of telehealth in HF on access, costs, and quality of care provided for securing permanent reimbursement for telemonitoring services.

SUMMARY

The goal of RPM in HF is to improve patient-reported health outcomes, reduce residual risk through the optimization of medical therapy, and enable timely interventions to reduce HF-related hospitalizations and mortality. To achieve these goals, it would be paramount for RPM interventions to emphasize monitoring parameters of devices, monitoring frequency, and adherence to the monitoring system. Having novel structured intervention strategies based on device data is critical for RPM's success. In the future, leveraging different technologies and devices at the right time across the HF disease spectrum can make a difference. Moving forward, the pace of innovation is going to continue while we gather data for remote monitoring devices, indicating a dynamic future for telemonitoring in HF.

CLINICS CARE POINTS

- Although earlier clinical trials did not show benefit of remote monitoring in patients with HF, recent trials that deployed advanced technologies, more efficient data monitoring, and prompt response to deviation of physiological parameters from preset thresholds have shown promise in reducing HF-related readmissions and mortality.

- Increase in body weight is an unreliable surrogate of cardiac congestion.

- CardioMEMS is the only FDA approved device for remote PA pressure monitoring for patients with NYHA II or III who have either been hospitalized for HF in the previous 12 months or have elevated natriuretic peptides.

- Clinical trials studying the benefit of a combination of invasive monitoring of cardiac filling pressures and vital signs are ongoing.

- HF clinics need to be restructured to integrate telemonitoring in their workflow.

DISCLOSURES

Dr A.J. Sauer reports receiving compensation from Abbott, Boston Scientific, Biotronik, Acorai, Story Health, General Prognostics, and Impulse Dynamics for advising, speaking, and performing research activities. Dr I. Mastoris has no relevant disclosures to this study. Dr K. Gupta has no relevant disclosures to this study.

REFERENCES

1. Takahashi EA, Schwamm LH, Adeoye OM, et al. An Overview of Telehealth in the Management of Cardiovascular Disease: A Scientific Statement From the American Heart Association. Circulation 2022; 146(25):e558–68.
2. Rosen D, McCall JD, Primack BA. Telehealth Protocol to Prevent Readmission Among High-Risk Patients With Congestive Heart Failure. Am J Med 2017;130(11):1326–30.
3. Inglis SC, Clark RA, Dierckx R, et al. Structured telephone support or non-invasive telemonitoring for patients with heart failure. Heart 2017;103(4): 255–7.
4. Mohebi R, Chen C, Ibrahim NE, et al. Cardiovascular Disease Projections in the United States Based on the 2020 Census Estimates. J Am Coll Cardiol 2022;80(6):565–78.
5. Roger VL. Epidemiology of Heart Failure: A Contemporary Perspective. Circ Res 2021;128(10):1421–34.
6. Van Nuys Karen E, Xie Zhiwen, Bryan Tysinger, et al. Goldman Dana P. Innovation in Heart Failure Treatment. JACC (J Am Coll Cardiol): Heart Fail 2018; 6(5):401–9.
7. Heidenreich PA, Albert NM, Allen LA, et al. Forecasting the Impact of Heart Failure in the United States. Circ Heart Fail 2013;6(3):606–19.
8. Virani SS, Alonso A, Benjamin EJ, et al. Heart Disease and Stroke Statistics-2020 Update: A Report From the American Heart Association. Circulation 2020;141(9):e139–596.
9. Khan MS, Sreenivasan J, Lateef N, et al. Trends in 30- and 90-Day Readmission Rates for Heart Failure. Circ Heart Fail 2021;14(4):e008335.
10. Super N. Medicare's Chronic Care Improvement Pilot Program: What Is Its Potential? https://hsrc. himmelfarb.gwu.edu/sphhs_centers_nhpf/128. 2004. Accessed January 16, 2023.
11. Krumholz HM, Merrill AR, Schone EM, et al. Patterns of hospital performance in acute myocardial infarction and heart failure 30-day mortality and readmission. Circ Cardiovasc Qual Outcomes 2009;2(5): 407–13.
12. And PP. Be it enacted by the Senate and House of Representatives of the United States of America in Congress assembled. 2010. https://www.congress. gov/111/plaws/publ148/PLAW-111publ148.pdf. Accessed January 16, 2023.
13. Goldberg LR, Piette JD, Walsh MN, et al. Randomized trial of a daily electronic home monitoring system in patients with advanced heart failure: the Weight Monitoring in Heart Failure (WHARF) trial. Am Heart J 2003;146(4):705–12.
14. Cleland John GF, Louis Amala A, Rigby Alan S, et al. null null. Noninvasive Home Telemonitoring for Patients With Heart Failure at High Risk of Recurrent

Admission and Death. J Am Coll Cardiol 2005; 45(10):1654–64.

15. Chaudhry SI, Barton B, Mattera J, et al. Randomized trial of Telemonitoring to Improve Heart Failure Outcomes (Tele-HF): study design. J Card Fail 2007; 13(9):709–14.

16. Soran OZ, Piña IL, Lamas GA, et al. A randomized clinical trial of the clinical effects of enhanced heart failure monitoring using a computer-based telephonic monitoring system in older minorities and women. J Card Fail 2008;14(9):711–7.

17. Mortara A, Pinna GD, Johnson P, et al. Home telemonitoring in heart failure patients: the HHH study (Home or Hospital in Heart Failure). Eur J Heart Fail 2009;11(3):312–8.

18. Chaudhry SI, Mattera JA, Curtis JP, et al. Telemonitoring in patients with heart failure. N Engl J Med 2010;363(24):2301–9.

19. Koehler F, Winkler S, Schieber M, et al. Impact of remote telemedical management on mortality and hospitalizations in ambulatory patients with chronic heart failure: the telemedical interventional monitoring in heart failure study. Circulation 2011; 123(17):1873–80.

20. Ong MK, Romano PS, Edgington S, et al. Effectiveness of Remote Patient Monitoring After Discharge of Hospitalized Patients With Heart Failure: The Better Effectiveness After Transition – Heart Failure (BEAT-HF) Randomized Clinical Trial. JAMA Intern Med 2016;176(3):310–8.

21. Heidenreich PA, Bozkurt B, Aguilar D, et al. 2022 AHA/ACC/HFSA Guideline for the Management of Heart Failure: A Report of the American College of Cardiology/American Heart Association Joint Committee on Clinical Practice Guidelines. Circulation 2022;145(18):e895–1032.

22. Koehler F, Koehler K, Deckwart O, et al. Efficacy of telemedical interventional management in patients with heart failure (TIM-HF2): a randomised, controlled, parallel-group, unmasked trial. Lancet 2018;392(10152):1047–57.

23. Desai AS. Home monitoring heart failure care does not improve patient outcomes: looking beyond telephone-based disease management. Circulation 2012;125(6):828–36.

24. Lewin J, Ledwidge M, O'Loughlin C, et al. Clinical deterioration in established heart failure: what is the value of BNP and weight gain in aiding diagnosis? Eur J Heart Fail 2005;7(6):953–7.

25. Chaudhry SI, Wang Y, Concato J, et al. Patterns of weight change preceding hospitalization for heart failure. Circulation 2007;116(14):1549–54.

26. Zhang J, Goode KM, Cuddihy PE, et al. Predicting hospitalization due to worsening heart failure using daily weight measurement: analysis of the Trans-European Network-Home-Care Management System (TEN-HMS) study. Eur J Heart Fail 2009;11(4):420–7.

27. Zile MR, Bennett TD, John Sutton M, et al. Transition from chronic compensated to acute decompensated heart failure: pathophysiological insights obtained from continuous monitoring of intracardiac pressures. Circulation 2008;118(14):1433–41.

28. Bourge Robert C, Abraham William T, Adamson Philip B, et al. Randomized Controlled Trial of an Implantable Continuous Hemodynamic Monitor in Patients With Advanced Heart Failure. J Am Coll Cardiol 2008;51(11):1073–9.

29. Teerlink JR. Learning the points of COMPASS-HF: assessing implantable hemodynamic monitoring in heart failure patients. J Am Coll Cardiol 2008; 51(11):1080–2.

30. Ritzema J, Troughton R, Melton I, et al. Physician-directed patient self-management of left atrial pressure in advanced chronic heart failure. Circulation 2010;121(9):1086–95.

31. Ritzema J, Melton IC, Richards AM, et al. Direct left atrial pressure monitoring in ambulatory heart failure patients: initial experience with a new permanent implantable device. Circulation 2007;116(25): 2952–9.

32. Maurer MS, Adamson PB, Costanzo MR, et al. Rationale and Design of the Left Atrial Pressure Monitoring to Optimize Heart Failure Therapy Study (LAPTOP-HF). J Card Fail 2015;21(6):479–88.

33. Abraham WT, Adamson PB, Costanzo MR, et al. Hemodynamic Monitoring in Advanced Heart Failure: Results from the LAPTOP-HF Trial. J Card Fail 2016;22(11):940.

34. Perl L, Meerkin D, D'amario D, et al. The V-LAP System for Remote Left Atrial Pressure Monitoring of Patients With Heart Failure: Remote Left Atrial Pressure Monitoring. J Card Fail 2022;28(6):963–72.

35. Adamson PB, Abraham WT, Aaron M, et al. CHAMPION trial rationale and design: the long-term safety and clinical efficacy of a wireless pulmonary artery pressure monitoring system. J Card Fail 2011; 17(1):3–10.

36. Abraham WT, Stevenson LW, Bourge RC, et al. Sustained efficacy of pulmonary artery pressure to guide adjustment of chronic heart failure therapy: complete follow-up results from the CHAMPION randomised trial. Lancet 2016;387(10017): 453–61.

37. Abraham WT, Adamson PB, Bourge RC, et al. Wireless pulmonary artery haemodynamic monitoring in chronic heart failure: a randomised controlled trial. Lancet 2011;377(9766):658–66.

38. Lindenfeld J, Zile MR, Desai AS, et al. Haemodynamic-guided management of heart failure (GUIDE-HF): a randomised controlled trial. Lancet 2021;398(10304):991–1001.

39. U.S. Food and Drug Administration. Premarket Approval (PMA) CardioMEMS HF System. 2022. https://www.accessdata.fda.gov/scripts/cdrh/cfdocs/

cfpma/pma.cfm?id=P100045S056. Accessed January 22, 2023.

40. Mullens W, Sharif F, Dupont M, et al. Digital health care solution for proactive heart failure management with the Cordella Heart Failure System: results of the SIRONA first-in-human study. Eur J Heart Fail 2020; 22(10):1912–9.

41. Sharif F, Rosenkranz S, Bartunek J, et al. Safety and efficacy of a wireless pulmonary artery pressure sensor: primary endpoint results of the SIRONA 2 clinical trial. ESC Heart Fail 2022;9(5):2862–72.

42. Guichard JL, Cowger JA, Chaparro SV, et al. Rationale and Design of the Proactive-HF Trial for Managing Patients With NYHA Class III Heart Failure by Using the Combined Cordella Pulmonary Artery Sensor and the Cordella Heart Failure System. J Card Fail 2022. https://doi.org/10.1016/j.cardfail. 2022.09.006.

43. PROACTIVE-HF IDE Trial Heart Failure NYHA Class III - Full Text View - Clinicaltrials.gov. Available at: https://clinicaltrials.gov/ct2/show/NCT04089059. Accessed January 22, 2023.

44. Yu CM, Wang L, Chau E, et al. Intrathoracic impedance monitoring in patients with heart failure: correlation with fluid status and feasibility of early warning preceding hospitalization. Circulation 2005;112(6): 841–8.

45. Abraham WT, Compton S, Haas G, et al. Superior Performance of Intrathoracic Impedance-Derived fluid Index versus Daily Weight monitoring in Heart Failure Patients: Results of the Fluid Accumulation Status Trial (FAST). J Card Fail 2009;15(9):813.

46. Mastoris I, Van Spall HGC, Sheldon SH, et al. Emerging Implantable-Device Technology for Patients at the Intersection of Electrophysiology and Heart Failure Interdisciplinary Care. J Card Fail 2022;28(6):991–1015.

47. Conraads VM, Tavazzi L, Santini M, et al. Sensitivity and positive predictive value of implantable intrathoracic impedance monitoring as a predictor of heart failure hospitalizations: the SENSE-HF trial. Eur Heart J 2011;32(18):2266–73.

48. Böhm M, Drexler H, Oswald H, et al. Fluid status telemedicine alerts for heart failure: a randomized controlled trial. Eur Heart J 2016;37(41):3154–63.

49. Burri H, da Costa A, Quesada A, et al. Risk stratification of cardiovascular and heart failure hospitalizations using integrated device diagnostics in patients with a cardiac resynchronization therapy defibrillator. Europace 2018;20(5):e69–77.

50. Morgan JM, Kitt S, Gill J, et al. Remote management of heart failure using implantable electronic devices. Eur Heart J 2017;38(30):2352–60.

51. Gardner RS, Singh JP, Stancak B, et al. HeartLogic Multisensor Algorithm Identifies Patients During Periods of Significantly Increased Risk of Heart Failure Events. Circ Heart Fail 2018;11(7):e004669.

52. Hernandez AF, Albert NM, Allen LA, et al. Multiple cArdiac seNsors for mAnaGEment of Heart Failure (MANAGE-HF) - Phase I Evaluation of the Integration and Safety of the HeartLogic Multisensor Algorithm in Patients With Heart Failure. J Card Fail 2022; 28(8):1245–54.

53. Sherazi S, Kutyifa V, McNitt S, et al. Prognostic Significance of Heart Rate Variability Among Patients Treated With Cardiac Resynchronization Therapy: MADIT-CRT (Multicenter Automatic Defibrillator Implantation Trial-Cardiac Resynchronization Therapy). JACC Clin Electrophysiol 2015;1(1–2):74–80.

54. Attia ZI, Harmon DM, Dugan J, et al. Prospective evaluation of smartwatch-enabled detection of left ventricular dysfunction. Nat Med 2022;28(12): 2497–503.

55. Bayoumy K, Gaber M, Elshafeey A, et al. Smart wearable devices in cardiovascular care: where we are and how to move forward. Nat Rev Cardiol 2021;18(8):581–99.

56. Ski CF, Thompson DR, Brunner-La Rocca HP. Putting AI at the centre of heart failure care. ESC Heart Fail 2020;7(5):3257–8.

57. Allen LA, Venechuk G, McIlvennan CK, et al. An Electronically Delivered Patient-Activation Tool for Intensification of Medications for Chronic Heart Failure With Reduced Ejection Fraction: The EPIC-HF Trial. Circulation 2021;143(5):427–37.

58. Walton A, Nahum-Shani I, Crosby L, et al. Optimizing Digital Integrated Care via Micro-Randomized Trials. Clin Pharmacol Ther 2018;104(1):53–8.

59. Ziaeian B, Fonarow GC. The Prevention of Hospital Readmissions in Heart Failure. Prog Cardiovasc Dis 2016;58(4):379–85.

60. Khan MS, Van Spall HGC. Effectiveness of Telemedicine Services After Hospitalization for Heart Failure: A Matter of Outcome?*. JACC (J Am Coll Cardiol): Heart Fail 2023. https://doi.org/10.1016/j.jchf.2022. 10.015.

61. Schwamm LH, Chumbler N, Brown E, et al. Recommendations for the Implementation of Telehealth in Cardiovascular and Stroke Care: A Policy Statement From the American Heart Association. Circulation 2017;135(7):e24–44.

62. Looking towards the future of telehealth in Medicare, evidence is needed. The White House; 2022. Available at: https://www.whitehouse.gov/ostp/news-updates/ 2022/11/10/looking-towards-the-future-of-telehealth-in-medicare-evidence-is-needed/. Accessed January 22, 2023.

Interventional Management of Atrial Fibrillation in the Chronic Heart Failure Population

Parin J. Patel, MD, FHRS[a],*, Asim S. Ahmed, DO, FHRS[b]

KEYWORDS

- Atrial fibrillation • Cardiac resynchronization therapy • Catheter ablation
- Conduction system pacing • Heart failure • Pulmonary vein isolation

KEY POINTS

- Atrial fibrillation (AF) and heart failure (HF) synergistically interact to exacerbate each other. However, treatment of one entity can greatly improve management of the other.
- Maintenance of sinus rhythm may be particularly important in the HF population. Non-pharmacologic approaches to AF management in HF are therefore increasingly attractive.
- Catheter ablation has good evidence for benefit in this population, but in those who cannot tolerate it, it would be reasonable to consider early adoption of AV junction ablation and cardiac resynchronization therapy device placement.

INTRODUCTION

Scope of the Problem

Atrial fibrillation (AF) is the most common arrhythmia worldwide, with a prevalence of 3% in the general adult population and 18% in those older than 85 years.[1] Furthermore, the population of AF patients is expected to almost double by 2030.[2] In addition, AF management in the United States accounts for over $20 billion yearly or about 1.5% of all health care expenditures, often requiring frequent office visits for medication titration and ER visits or hospitalizations for acute exacerbations.[3]

The burden of heart failure (HF) is also high, but advances in HF management have resulted in a declining incidence.[4] The combination of both established and new pharmacologic therapies including beta blockers, angiotensin converting enzyme-inhibitors, angiotensin receptor-neprilysin inhibitors, mineralocorticoid antagonists, and sodium/glucose cotransporter-2 Inhibitors (the so-called "quadruple therapy") shows promise in reducing HF hospitalization, morbidity, and mortality. However, improving survival increases prevalence, and HF nevertheless continues to be a common reason for hospitalization, affecting a similar 3% of the population but composing 8% of the health care burden in the United States.[5,6]

Cause and Consequence

There is a synergy between AF and HF on multiple levels. The symptoms of each condition include dyspnea on exertion, shortness of breath, exercise intolerance, and volume overload. In addition, HF with mid-range or preserved ejection fraction accounts for half of all HF hospitalizations and can both predispose to and be exacerbated by AF.[7,8] In addition, HF and AF share common risk factors such as hypertension, sleep apnea, obesity, diabetes, and coronary artery disease. AF can also be a direct cause of HF, especially in cases of

[a] Department of Cardiac Electrophysiology, Ascension St. Vincent Heart Center, 8333 Naab Road #400, Indianapolis, IN 46260, USA; [b] Department of Cardiac Electrophysiology, Ascension Sacred Heart Cardiology, 5151 North 9th Avenue #200, Pensacola, FL 32504, USA
* Corresponding author.
E-mail address: parin.patel@ascension.org
Twitter: @drparinpatel (P.J.P.); @AsimAhmedEP (A.S.A.)

Heart Failure Clin 20 (2024) 15–28
https://doi.org/10.1016/j.hfc.2023.05.009
1551-7136/24/© 2023 Elsevier Inc. All rights reserved.

tachycardia-induced cardiomyopathy, one of the few completely reversible causes of HF. However, even when adequately rate controlled, loss of atrial kick during AF can reduce cardiac output by up to 30%, which may be enough to push a chronically stable HF patient into an acute exacerbation.[9] On the other hand, chronically higher filling pressure with systolic or diastolic HF, mitral annular dilation, and functional mitral regurgitation are all risk factors for AF. It is often difficult to tease out cause and effect in cases of overlap, and so parallel treatment strategies are frequently warranted.

Old is Not Gold

Thus, the maintenance of sinus rhythm may be particularly important in the HF population. However, two major trials have historically turned popular opinion against sinus rhythm in the HF population: AFFIRM-HF and AF-congestive heart failure (CHF).[10,11] Both trials rely on data from approaches almost 2 decades old and involve drugs that increased mortality in the rhythm control group.[12] Unfortunately, most medications for sinus rhythm maintenance have contraindications in HF and renal impairment or interaction with life-prolonging medicines. Most experienced cardiologists hesitate to use class I antiarrhythmic agents in those with structurally abnormal hearts based on the CAST trial.[13] Furthermore, ANDROMEDA showed evidence of harm with dronedarone in the HF population,[14] and using sotalol at high doses may increase mortality in the coronary disease population[15] or limit the use of evidence-based beta blockers. Amiodarone is often the only drug remaining, but lessons from AFFIRM are still fresh: sinus rhythm had a mortality benefit, but this was offset by toxic effects of amiodarone.[12]

Non-pharmacologic approaches to AF management in HF are therefore increasingly attractive. The authors review here recent advances in catheter ablation (CA) of AF as well as the "pace-and-ablate" strategy of pacemaker implantation and subsequent AV node ablation (**Fig. 1**).

REVIEW OF CONTEMPORANEOUS DATA
Ancient History to the Recent Past

Ancient Egyptians held a remarkably accurate notion of pulmonary edema, cardiac hypertrophy, and congestive HF.[16,17] Chinese doctors from 2600 BCE described peripheral edema in the "Yellow Emperor's Classic of Internal Medicine."[18] Understanding of the pulse and rhythm of the heart would come later, during the time of Galen in the second century.[19]

Understanding the interplay between AF and HF would take millennia, but the maintenance of sinus rhythm by CA in the HF population is not an entirely new concept. Haissaguerre and colleagues presented positive findings in a group of 58 patients with HF undergoing CA in 2004.[20] In fact, several older reviews comprehensively address the sparse data on the subject.[21,22] Meta-analyses have also tackled the subject, showing an overall benefit of CA.[23–27] However, this article focuses on more recent data from randomized controlled trials, starting with the first large-scale trial of CA of AF in HF patients: Catheter Ablation for Atrial Fibrillation with Heart Failure (CASTLE-AF).[28] (**Table 1**)

Timeline for Catheter Ablation of Atrial Fibrillation in Heart Failure

In this landmark trial, the CASTLE investigators conducted a multicenter, open-label, randomized controlled trial comparing medical management of AF against CA of AF from 2008 to 2016. Inclusion criteria were patients with clinical HF (worse than NYHA class 1), ejection fraction $\leq$ 35%, implantable cardioverter defibrillator (ICD), and any type of AF (paroxysmal or persistent) failing antiarrhythmic drug therapy (for inefficacy, side effects, or patient choice). Randomization included 363 subjects assigned 1:1 to CA or standard of care, but both groups received a 5 week run-in period uptitrating optimal medical therapy as tolerated. The ablation strategy was operator dependent, but all cases involved at least pulmonary vein isolation (PVI).

The primary outcome was composite all-cause mortality or hospitalization for HF. With mean 3 years of follow-up, there was a significant difference in the primary outcome between the ablation and medical therapy group: HR 0.62 (0.43–0.87, P = .006). On subgroup analysis, there was lower rate of all-cause mortality (13% vs 25%), HF hospitalization (21% vs 36%), cardiovascular (CV) death (11% vs 22%), and CV hospitalization (36% vs 48%). There was no difference in all-cause hospitalization or stroke. After CA, median improvement in EF was 7% in those with paroxysmal AF and 10% in those who were persistent.

Another study performed concurrently with CASTLE was Catheter Ablation versus Best Medical Therapy in Patients with Persistent Atrial Fibrillation and Congestive Heart Failure (AMICA) by Kuck and colleagues.[29] In this multicenter, open-label, randomized controlled trial, a similar HF population with persistent or long-standing persistent AF was randomized to CA or medical therapy. The primary outcome was change in baseline LVEF, which was estimated to increase by 15% in the CA arm and 5% in the medical therapy

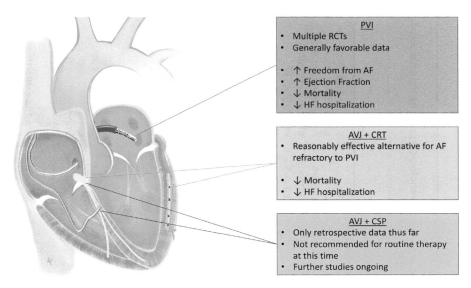

PVI
• Multiple RCTs
• Generally favorable data

• ↑ Freedom from AF
• ↑ Ejection Fraction
• ↓ Mortality
• ↓ HF hospitalization

AVJ + CRT
• Reasonably effective alternative for AF refractory to PVI

• ↓ Mortality
• ↓ HF hospitalization

AVJ + CSP
• Only retrospective data thus far
• Not recommended for routine therapy at this time
• Further studies ongoing

Fig. 1. Non-pharmacologic approaches to management of atrial fibrillation in patients with heart failure. The central figure depicts a summary of current and novel strategies for management of atrial fibrillation in patients with heart failure. Data regarding percutaneous catheter ablation approaches focusing on pulmonary vein isolation as the mainstay of interventional therapy are depicted in blue (summary box and catheter). Data for bionic therapy consisting of cardiac resynchronization and accompanying atrioventricular junction ablation are depicted with a green box and green lead entering the coronary sinus and exiting on the lateral aspect of the left ventricle. Last, the limited data encompassing utilization of conduction system pacing in lieu of traditional cardiac resynchronization therapy with the aforementioned atrioventricular junction ablation are depicted via the orange box and orange lead entering the conduction system.

arm (numbers drawn largely from the CAMERA-MRI trial: 18% vs 4.4%).[30] This was a negative trial, with no difference in primary outcome at 1 year follow-up (8.8% vs 7.3%, $P = .36$). Although secondary endpoints were not powered, there was significantly more sinus rhythm at 1 year follow-up and lower AF burden in the CA group.

A major criticism of AMICA is that the investigators guessed wrong on the primary endpoint. CASTLE, which included more subjects, showed a more modest improvement in EF of only 10%. Recalculating power analysis in AMICA using 10% increase in EF shows that they would have needed 840 subjects to show a difference. Furthermore, the 7.3% increase in EF in the control group was higher than expected, showing great efficacy of pharmacologic therapy for this endpoint. Hard endpoints such as CV hospitalization or death from CASTLE are more appealing. Furthermore, CASTLE specifically biased away from antiarrhythmic drug use, as more than half of those getting CA failed amiodarone; more than one-third AMICA patients who got CA remained on amiodarone. This reinforces the possible toxic effect of amiodarone in this population.

Another contemporaneous trial of CA in CHF was Ablation versus Amiodarone for Treatment of Persistent Atrial Fibrillation in Patients with Congestive Heart Failure and an Implanted Device (AATAC) by Di Biase and colleagues.[31] This was again a multicenter, open-label, parallel-group, randomized trial of patients with persistent AF, prior ICD, class II or III HF, EF less than 40 assigned CA or amiodarone. More aggressive ablation was done in this study, with at least PVI, but recommendation to perform posterior wall isolation, superior vena cava (SVC) isolation, and any additional non-PV triggers or linear lesions per operator discretion. Primary endpoint was AF recurrence, with minimum of 2 year follow-up.

AATAC met the primary endpoint with 70% of CA patients being arrhythmia free compared with 34% on amiodarone ($P < .001$). The CA group also had lower unplanned hospitalization (31% vs 58%) and all-cause mortality (8% vs 18%). EF improved by 8.3% after ablation compared with 5.0% after amiodarone ($P = .02$), and several quality of life metrics were better after CA (6MWD and MLFHQ).

More Recent Trials with Catheter Ablation for Atrial Fibrillation in Heart Failure

The previously referenced clinical trials are the largest randomized trials powered for hard outcomes examining the role of CA for AF in the HF

Table 1
Multicenter randomized controlled trials comparing varying strategies of catheter ablation versus medical therapy in chronological order based on date of publication

Name	Sample Size	Population	Medication Strategy	Ablation Strategy	Primary Endpoint	Results	Context
AATAC 2016	203	PeAF, ICD, NYHA II or III HF, EF < 40	Amiodarone	PVI ± PWI ± CFAE	AF recurrence	Significant increase in freedom from AF in CA group compared with amiodarone	CA group had lower unplanned hospitalization and all-cause mortality and higher EF improvement and quality of life compared with amiodarone
CASTLE-AF 2018	363	NYHA ≥ II, EF ≤ 35%, ICD, and PAF or PeAF failing AAD	Rate or rhythm control	PVI ± linear ablation ± CFAE	Composite all-cause mortality or HF hospitalization	Significant reduction in composite of death and HF hospitalization in CA group	After CA, median EF improvement of 7% in PAF and 10% in PeAF
AMICA 2019	140	HF with PeAF or longstanding PeAF	Rate or rhythm control	PVI ± additional targets per operator discretion	Change in baseline EF	No difference in primary outcome	Overestimation of primary endpoint (underpowered for EF improvement and competing with EF improvement from medical therapy) More than one-third of CA arm remained on amiodarone (known toxic effects)

	N	Inclusion	Intervention	Ablation	Primary Endpoint	Result	Comments
CABANA 2019	2204	PAF or PeAF within previous 6 mo	Rate or rhythm control	PVI ± additional targets per operator discretion	Composite of all-cause mortality, disabling stroke, serious bleeding, or cardiac arrest	Intention to treat analysis failed to meet significance of the primary endpoint	Poor enrollment. 30% crossover between arms. The as treated analysis showed significantly lower risk of primary endpoint and secondary endpoint of death or CV mortality in the CA arm
EAST-AFNET 4 2020	2789	PAF diagnosed within previous 1 y ± 1 or more cardiovascular risk factors	Rate or rhythm control, which could include ablation	PVI	Composite CV death, stroke, or CV hospitalization	Significant reduction of primary endpoint in early rhythm control arm	HF hospitalization was not significantly different, likely reflecting the lack of HF population
CABANA HF 2021	778	NYHA II or higher, irrespective of EF. 9.3% of patients had EF < 40%, and 11.7% had EF 40%–50%.	Rate or rhythm control	PVI ± additional targets per operator discretion	Composite of death, serious stroke, bleeding, or cardiac arrest	Significantly lower in the CA arm compared with drug therapy. All-cause mortality, death or HF hospitalization, and AF burden also lower	Remarkable despite high crossover rate with almost 10% of ablation patients not receiving ablation, and 22% of drug therapy patients receiving ablation

(continued on next page)

Table 1
(continued)

Name	Sample Size	Population	Medication Strategy	Ablation Strategy	Primary Endpoint	Results	Context
RAFT-AF 2022	411	High-burden AF ($\geq$ 4 episodes in the prior 6 mo), NYHA II-III with any EF, elevated NT-proBNP with or without HF hospitalization in the prior 9 mo	Rate control	PVI for PAF and of PVI $\pm$ linear ablation, CFAE, and PWI per operator discretion for PeAF	Composite of death or HF event (hospitalization, acute clinic visit with medicine changes or IV diuretic administration)	Primary outcome did not meet statistical significance but was less common in the CA arm compared with rate control. EF improvement significantly higher after CA	Stopped early for futility due to limited enrollment and a lower than expected event rate. Higher AAD use in CA arm could possibly explain mitigated efficacy for primary endpoint

Abbreviations: AAD, anti-arrhythmic drugs; CA, catheter ablation; CFAE, complex fractionated atrial electrograms; EF, ejection fraction; HF, heart failure; ICD, implantable cardioverter defibrillator; NYHA, New York Heart Association; PAF, paroxysmal atrial fibrillation; PeAF, persistent atrial fibrillation; PVI, pulmonary vein isolation; PWI, posterior wall isolation.

population. Several smaller studies have confirmed similar benefits tweaking parameters or inclusion criteria (eg, cryoablation, diastolic HF).[32,33] However, there are several substudies from larger recent trials to note.

The Catheter Ablation versus Antiarrhythmic Drug Therapy for Atrial Fibrillation (CABANA) trial was a multicenter, open-label, randomized controlled trial with a primary endpoint of composite all-cause mortality, disabling stroke, serious bleeding, or cardiac arrest.[34] Because of poor enrollment (most enrolling doctors had strong opinions about utility of CA), the primary endpoint was modified midway through the study period. In addition, there was almost 30% crossover into the ablation arm. A total of 2204 patients were enrolled (about half of the initially powered population) and the intention to treat analysis failed to meet significance of the primary endpoint, though there may have been a trend toward significance if enrollment continued. The as-treated analysis showed significantly lower risk of the primary endpoint in the CA arm (HR 0.73, $P = .046$) as well as secondary endpoint of death or CV mortality (HR 0.83, $P = .002$). The ablation strategy once again included PVI and additional ablation per operator discretion, but the actual ablation strategies used in the trial have not been published to date.

Although subgroup analysis for a trial that fails to meet the primary endpoint has its statistical drawbacks,[35] the CABANA investigators have nevertheless presented strong physiology-based mechanistic justifications for doing so. One such analysis is the CABANA-HF trial, examining the subpopulation with clinical HF NYHA class II and higher, irrespective of EF.[36] The primary outcome of death, stroke, serious bleeding, or cardiac arrest was statistically significantly less common in the CA arm compared with drug therapy (HR 0.64, CI 0.41–0.99).

This was a remarkable finding, given that there remained a high crossover rate with almost 10% of ablation patients not getting an ablation, and 22% of drug therapy patients getting an ablation. When reanalyzed as on-treatment, the primary endpoint findings were even more robust (HR 0.58, CI 0.37–0.90). All-cause mortality and death or HF hospitalization were also less likely with CA (HR 0.50; HR 0.59). At all time points, using both proprietary AF monitors (42%) or standard of care monitoring, AF burden was significantly lower in the CA arm, examined using various metrics such as total AF burden, time to first AF, and presence of AF during a clinic visit. Importantly, symptom improvement was robust using both AFEQT (Atrial Fibrillation Effect on Quality of Life) and MAFSI (Mayo Atrial Fibrillation-Specific Symptom

Inventory) frequency scoring. Unfortunately, no specific HF outcomes other than HF hospitalization were examined; this is likely because inclusion criteria only required clinical HF (not EF cutoff), and baseline EF was missing in 27% of the population.

A more recent trial examined early intervention for maintenance of sinus rhythm in all comers with a new diagnosis of AF: EAST-AFNET 4 (Early Rhythm-Control Therapy in Patients with Atrial Fibrillation).[37] Although not specific for ablation, this was an international, multicenter, investigator-initiated, parallel-group, open-label trial of those with early AF (<1 year from diagnosis) and CV risk factors randomized to rate or rhythm control, which could include ablation. While not strictly an HF population either, the investigators were clearly interested in this population, spending half of the introduction in their manuscript examining the nexus of AF and HF. They conclude that because rhythm control had been mostly drug-induced in past trials, they wanted to perform a contemporary study of all rhythm control strategies. Consistent with real-world practice, CA was indeed performed in 20% of rhythm control subjects (and 7% of the control arm), though the ablation strategy is not well-defined.

The primary outcome of composite CV death, stroke, or CV hospitalization was reduced in the early rhythm control arm (HR 0.79, CI 0.66–0.94, $P = .005$). HF hospitalization was not significantly different (HR 0.81, CI 0.65–1.02), and increased EF was statistically significant (HR 0.23, −0.46–0.91) but not clinically significant (1.5% vs 0.8%). The lack of significantly improved HF outcomes no doubt reflects the lack of enrichment for an HF population. It should be noted that almost 30% of the enrolled subjects had clinical HF, and we eagerly await the planned substudy of EAST-AF-HF that is likely in the works.

Another noteworthy AF and HF trial is the Randomized Ablation-Based Rhythm-Control versus Rate-Control Trial in Patients with Heart Failure and Atrial Fibrillation.[38] RAFT-AF was a multicenter, open-label, randomized controlled trial in patients with high burden AF (defined as $\geq$ 4 episodes in the prior 6 month) and NYHA class 2 to 3 symptoms with any EF. Elevated NT-proBNP with or without HF hospitalization in the prior 9 month was also an entry requirement, adjusted for the presence of AF. Ablation was PVI only for paroxysmal AF patients and combinations of PVI plus lines, CFAE ablation, and posterior wall isolation per operator discretion for persistent AF patients. Rate control patients received uptitration of beta blockers, calcium channel blockers, or digoxin targeting resting HR less than 80 or 6MWT HR < 110 bpm. Unlike prior studies such as AFFIRM, oral anticoagulation was recommended for both arms irrespective of long-term outcomes.

The lofty primary outcome was a composite of death or HF event (hospitalization, acute clinic visit with medicine changes, or IV diuretic administration). Unfortunately, like CABANA, this trial was plagued by more limited enrollment and a lower than expected event rate, so an interim analysis recommended stopping early for futility after enrollment of 411 patients (out of a planned 600 patients). Incredibly, in light of CABANA, there was absolutely no crossover from the rate control arm to the ablation arm and only 3% non-ablation in the CA group.

The primary outcome did not meet statistical significance but was less common in the CA arm compared with rate control (24% vs 33%, HR 0.71, CI 0.49–1.03, P = .06). However, improvement in EF was significantly higher after CA (10.1% vs 3.8%, P = .017). This is especially remarkable given that 40% of subjects had EF $\geq$ 45% at baseline. Although severely underpowered, the improvement in primary outcome as well as key secondary outcomes (6-minute walk test distance [6MWTD], AFEQT, Minnesota Living with Heart Failure Questionnaire [MLHFQ]) seemed to be greater in the EF less than 45 group. It also seemed that the ablation was less useful in long-standing persistent AF and more helpful in paroxysmal and early-persistent AF, a finding echoed in CABANA but opposite to CASTLE. Fewer patients in the control arm were on antiarrhythmic medications because a strategy of rate control was adopted (6% vs 22%); the higher antiarrhythmic drug usage in CA patients could explain mitigated efficacy for the primary endpoint. In addition, there was an almost 50% complication rate in the ablation arm, much higher than the 7% found in CABANA. Finally, a whopping 30% of patients in the rate control arm received atrio-ventricular (AV) junction ablation and pacemaker placement, which may be the final common endpoint of a strictly rate control strategy when there is no crossover to rhythm control. The investigators did not disclose how many patients received cardiac resynchronization (CRT).

Bionic Therapy for Atrial Fibrillation in Heart Failure

The broader therapy of CRT is underused, but increasing in incidence, for advanced HF patients.[39] However, the original trials for CRT excluded those in AF at the time of enrollment.[40] Nevertheless, almost half of patients in AMICA and 15% (or about half of reduced-EF patients)

in RAFT-AF had CRT at some point during the trial.

This leads us to examine evidence for improved AF outcomes with CRT. Indeed, subsequent subgroup analyses of CRT trials show benefit of CRT compared with medical therapy even in those with incident AF.[38,41] In addition, CRT reduces the risk of incident AF, and in those who develop AF, CRT reduces mortality.[42] The data favor continued use of CRT in appropriate AF-HF patients (low EF, wide QRS with left-sided involvement, NYHA>1), though efforts at adequate rate control are especially important to allow a threshold effect of 95% to 98% biventricular pacing[43,44] (**Table 2**).

Optimal Strategy for Bionic Therapy

Thus, CRT is an option in the appropriate AF-HF patient. However, it is not yet known when during the progression of HF treatment CA should be offered versus CRT. If cardiomyopathy is thought to result from uncontrolled AF, CA is likely appropriate first. The question of CA or CRT + atrioventricular junction (AVJ) ablation was examined in the Pulmonary-Vein Isolation for Atrial Fibrillation in Patients with Heart Failure (PABA-CHF) trial.[45]

In this prospective, multicenter, open-label trial, patients with EF $\leq$ 40% and NYHA 2 to 3 symptoms who also had drug-refractory, symptomatic AF were randomized to PVI or AVJ ablation + CRT. The primary endpoint was a composite of EF, 6MWTD and MLWHF score, a common HF/ICD endpoint. The ablation strategy was again PVI plus additional ablation per operator discretion.

CA was superior to AVJ ablation + CRT-D at 6 month follow-up, with improvement in EF of 76% versus 25% (P < .001) and mean increase in EF of 8.8% versus −1% (P < .001); almost 100 m increase in 6MWTD vs no change (P < .001); and better MLWHF score (30% change vs no change, P < .001). PABA-CHF showed similar results to CASTLE-AF, with a better improvement in outcomes in those with non-paroxysmal AF. A number of curiosities abound in this trial, however. As follow-up EF remained below 40% in the CA arm, it was unclear how many CA patients eventually received ICD therapy. In addition, the rate of CRT response (25%) was far below what would be expected (nearly 70%) from prior CRT trials.[40,42–44] Nevertheless, PABA-CHF confirms that it may be reasonable to consider at least one or two attempts at CA of AF before committing a stable HF patient to AVJ ablation and CRT.

Occasionally, however, those with severely symptomatic HF or those with longstanding

Table 2
Trials using bionic therapy strategies in patients with atrial fibrillation refractory to rate and rhythm control therapies

Name	Sample Size	Design	Population	Intervention	Ablation Strategy	Primary Endpoint	Results	Context
PABA-HF 2008	81	Multicenter, open-label RCT	EF ≤ 40%, NYHA II-III, symptomatic AF refractory to AAD	Randomized to PVI or AVJ ablation ± CRT	PVI ± additional ablation per operator discretion or AVJ ablation + CRT	Composite of EF, 6MWTD and MLWHF score	CA was superior to AVJ ablation + CRT	EF remained below 40% in the CA arm; it was unclear how many CA patients eventually received ICD therapy Rate of CRT response (25%) was far below what would be expected (nearly 70%) from prior CRT trials[40,42–44]
APAF-CRT 2021	133	Multicenter, open-label RCT	Permanent AF and severely symptomatic HF with narrow baseline QRS	Randomized to aggressive rate control or AVJ ablation and CRT	AVJ ablation + CRT	All-cause mortality	Stopped early for efficacy due to meeting primary endpoint Secondary endpoint of HF hospitalization was also lower in ablation arm	Higher amiodarone and digoxin use in the control arm, which could bias results against medical therapy No change in outcome when stratified by EF or presence of ICD

(continued on next page)

Table 2
(continued)

Name	Sample Size	Design	Population	Intervention	Ablation Strategy	Primary Endpoint	Results	Context
Conduction system pacing vs conventional pacing in patients undergoing atrioventricular node ablation: Non-randomized, on-treatment comparison (2022)	223	Nonrandomized, retrospective analysis	Patients undergoing AVJ ablation for refractory AF at Geisinger Health System between January 2015 and October 2020	CP or CSP per operator discretion	AVJ ablation ± either CP or CSP	Combination of time to death or HF hospitalization	Significant reduction of primary endpoint in CSP arm compared with CP No reduction in secondary outcomes of time to death and HF hospitalization between arms	Baseline EF was significantly different in the two groups (47% in CSP vs 36% in CP)
Biventricular vs Conduction System Pacing after Atrioventricular Node Ablation in Heart Failure Patients with Atrial Fibrillation (2022)	50	Single-center, observational, retrospective analysis	All consecutive patients undergoing pacemaker implantation in conjunction with AVJ ablation for refractory AF between May 2015 and January 2022	CP or CSP per operator discretion	AVJ ablation ± either CP or CSP	NYHA class and EF	Improvement in NYHA class and EF with CSP compared with CRT	Only 13 patients received at CRT and this response rate was again lower than what would be expected from prior CRT trials[40,42–44]

Abbreviations: 6MWTD, 6-minute walk test distance, AVJ, atrioventricular junction; CP, conventional pacing, CRT, cardiac resynchronization therapy; CSP, conduction system pacing, MLWHF, Minnesota Living with Heart Failure; PVI, pulmonary vein isolation, RCT, randomized controlled trial.

persistent AF (who have a lower likelihood of ablation success) may not be good candidates for CA.[38] This population was studied in the AV junction ablation and CRT for patients with permanent AF and narrow QRS (APAF-CRT) trial.[46]

This was a multicenter, open-label, trial randomizing patients with permanent AF and severely symptomatic HF with narrow baseline QRS to aggressive rate control or AVJ ablation and CRT. Per the RACE 2 trial, target resting HR in the control arm was less than 110 bpm.[47] The primary endpoint was all-cause mortality. The trial met its primary endpoint and was stopped early for efficacy (11% vs 29%, $P = .004$). Furthermore, the secondary endpoint of HF hospitalization was also lower in the intervention arm (HR 0.4, CI 0.22–0.73). Curiously, there was no change in outcome when stratified by EF or presence of ICD. In addition, there was more amiodarone and digoxin use in the control arm, which could bias results against medicines. However, if we believe the lack of EF interaction, the results remain valid in both reduced- and preserved-EF populations of HF.

New Kid on the Block

All of the CRT trials in AF presented thus far included those getting conventional left ventricular pacing leads implanted via the coronary sinus. We would be remiss to ignore a large and burgeoning field of interest when considering resynchronization therapy: conduction system pacing (CSP), or placement of the ventricular pacing to engage the native conduction system resulting in a narrow QRS.

Initial excitement over His bundle area pacing leads cooled after long-term outcomes showed increased thresholds (requiring more frequent battery changes) and eventual loss of His bundle capture (due to distal block or local tissue changes).[48] The field has increasingly moved toward deep septal pacing to engage the left bundle branch area, with QRS complexes that rival the native, narrow QRS.[49]

Although large-scale, randomized controlled trials are lacking, the initial experience at a high-volume center showed marginally favorable outcomes of CSP compared with traditional CRT after AVN ablation in a non-randomized, retrospective analysis where operator discretion was used to determine treatment.[50] It is hardly a fair comparison, as baseline EF was significantly different in the two groups (47% vs 36%). Another retrospective study using historical controls found no difference in HF outcomes.[51] Another smaller study of only 50 consecutive patients receiving CSP versus traditional CRT after AVN ablation showed improvement in NYHA class and EF ($P = .008$

and .041, respectively) with CSP compared with CRT.[52] However, only 13 patients received CRT and this response rate was again lower than what would be expected from prior CRT trials.

At this juncture, the data do not support the routine use of CSP in lieu of traditional CRT when making decisions about pacemaker therapy in the AF-HF population. However, we welcome future randomized trials asking this important question, such as the Conduction System Pacing versus Biventricular Pacing After Atrioventricular Node Ablation in Heart Failure Patients with Symptomatic Atrial Fibrillation and Narrow QRS (CONDUCT-AF) trial (NCT05467163).

PARTING THOUGHTS

AF and HF synergistically interact to exacerbate each other. However, it is also a two-way street, and treatment of one entity can greatly improve management of the other. Though historically, permissive medical therapy was the mainstay of AF management in the HF population, recent data strongly favor early, often invasive, intervention for AF to reduce hard HF outcomes. It seems that intervening earlier in the time course of AF, though still not excluding persistent AF from treatment, may have more pronounced effects. CA has good evidence for benefit in this population, but in those who cannot tolerate it, it would be reasonable to consider early adoption of AV junction ablation and CRT device placement.

CLINICS CARE POINTS

- Atrial fibrillation (AF) and heart failure (HF) are coexisting pathologies that share common risk factors and serve both as a cause and consequence to one another.

- Catheter ablation (CA) via pulmonary vein isolation and maintenance of sinus rhythm may significantly decrease the severity of HF and reduce HF hospitalizations

- Bionic therapy with traditional cardiac resynchronization therapy (CRT) in conjunction with atrioventricular junction (AVJ) ablation is an effective alternative for patients who remain recalcitrant to medical therapy and pulmonary vein isolation.

- Although currently available literature does not support the routine use of conduction system pacing as an alternative to CRT in combination with AVJ ablation, ongoing studies may potentially change this.

DISCLOSURE

Dr P.J. Patel reports consulting fees from Boston Scientific and Biosense Webster. Dr A.S Ahmed reports none.

REFERENCES

1. Williams BA, Chamberlain AM, Blankenship JC, et al. Trends in Atrial Fibrillation Incidence Rates Within an Integrated Health Care Delivery System, 2006 to 2018. JAMA Netw Open 2020;3(8): e2014874.

2. Miyasaka Y, Barnes ME, Gersh BJ, et al. Secular trends in incidence of atrial fibrillation in Olmsted County, Minnesota, 1980 to 2000, and implications on the projections for future prevalence. Circulation 2006;114(2):119–25. Erratum in: Circulation. 2006 Sep 12;114(11):e498. PMID: 16818816.

3. Kim MH, Johnston SS, Chu BC, et al. Estimation of total incremental health care costs in patients with atrial fibrillation in the United States. Circ Cardiovasc Qual Outcomes 2011;4(3):313–20.

4. Khera R, Pandey A, Ayers CR, et al. Contemporary Epidemiology of Heart Failure in Fee-For-Service Medicare Beneficiaries Across Healthcare Settings. Circ Heart Fail 2017;10(11):e004402.

5. Heidenreich PA, Albert NM, Allen LA, et al. American Heart Association Advocacy Coordinating Committee; Council on Arteriosclerosis, Thrombosis and Vascular Biology; Council on Cardiovascular Radiology and Intervention; Council on Clinical Cardiology; Council on Epidemiology and Prevention; Stroke Council. Forecasting the impact of heart failure in the United States: a policy statement from the American Heart Association. Circ Heart Fail 2013; 6(3):606–19.

6. Lesyuk W, Kriza C, Kolominsky-Rabas P. Cost-of-illness studies in heart failure: a systematic review 2004-2016. BMC Cardiovasc Disord 2018;18(1):74.

7. Kotecha D, Lam CS, Van Veldhuisen DJ, et al. Heart Failure With Preserved Ejection Fraction and Atrial Fibrillation: Vicious Twins. J Am Coll Cardiol 2016; 68(20):2217–28.

8. Noseworthy PA, Gersh BJ, Kent DM, et al. Atrial fibrillation ablation in practice: assessing CABANA generalizability. Eur Heart J 2019;40(16):1257–64.

9. Harada D, Asanoi H, Noto T, et al. The Impact of Deep Y Descent on Hemodynamics in Patients With Heart Failure and Preserved Left Ventricular Systolic Function. Front Cardiovasc Med 2021;8: 770923.

10. Wyse DG, Waldo AL, DiMarco JP, et al. Atrial Fibrillation Follow-up Investigation of Rhythm Management (AFFIRM) Investigators. A comparison of rate control and rhythm control in patients with atrial fibrillation. N Engl J Med 2002;347(23):1825–33.

11. Roy D, Talajic M, Nattel S, et al. Atrial Fibrillation and Congestive Heart Failure Investigators. Rhythm control versus rate control for atrial fibrillation and heart failure. N Engl J Med 2008;358(25):2667–77.

12. Corley SD, Epstein AE, DiMarco JP, et al. AFFIRM Investigators. Relationships between sinus rhythm, treatment, and survival in the Atrial Fibrillation Follow-Up Investigation of Rhythm Management (AFFIRM) Study. Circulation 2004;109(12):1509–13.

13. Echt DS, Liebson PR, Mitchell LB, et al. Mortality and Morbidity in Patients Receiving Encainide, Flecainide, or Placebo — The Cardiac Arrhythmia Suppression Trial. N Engl J Med 1991;324:781–8.

14. Køber L, Torp-Pedersen C, McMurray JJ, et al, Dronedarone Study Group. Increased mortality after dronedarone therapy for severe heart failure. N Engl J Med 2008;358(25):2678–87. Erratum in: N Engl J Med. 2010 Sep 30;363(14):1384. PMID: 18565860.

15. Waldo AL, Camm AJ, deRuyter H, et al. Effect of d-sotalol on mortality in patients with left ventricular dysfunction after recent and remote myocardial infarction. The SWORD Investigators. Survival With Oral d-Sotalol. Lancet 1996;348(9019):7–12. Erratum in: Lancet 1996 Aug 10;348(9024):416. PMID: 8691967.

16. Bianucci R, Loynes RD, Sutherland ML, et al. Forensic Analysis Reveals Acute Decompensation of Chronic Heart Failure in a 3500-Year-Old Egyptian Dignitary. J Forensic Sci 2016;61(5):1378–81.

17. Ferrari R. The story of the heartbeat, I: part I—heart rate: the rhythm of life. Eur Heart J 2012;33(1):4–5.

18. Freis ED. Historical development of antihypertensive treatment. In: Laragh J, Brenner BM, editors. Hypertension: pathophysiology, diagnosis, and management. eds 2nd ed. New York: Raven Press Ltd; 1995. p. 2741–51.

19. Harris CRS. The heart and the vascular system in ancient Greek medicine, from alcmaeon to galen. Oxford: Clarendon Press; 1973.

20. Hsu LF, Jaïs P, Sanders P, et al. Catheter ablation for atrial fibrillation in congestive heart failure. N Engl J Med 2004;351(23):2373–83.

21. Liang JJ, Callans DJ. Ablation for Atrial Fibrillation in Heart Failure with Reduced Ejection Fraction. Card Fail Rev 2010;4(1):33–7.

22. Anter E, Jessup M, Callans DJ. Atrial fibrillation and heart failure: treatment considerations for a dual epidemic. Circulation 2009;119(18):2516–25.

23. Turagam MK, Garg J, Whang W, et al. Catheter Ablation of Atrial Fibrillation in Patients With Heart Failure: A Meta-analysis of Randomized Controlled Trials. Ann Intern Med 2019;170(1):41–50. Erratum in: Ann Intern Med. 2019 May 7;170(9):668-669.

24. AlTurki A, Proietti R, Dawas A, et al. Catheter ablation for atrial fibrillation in heart failure with reduced ejection fraction: a systematic review and meta-

analysis of randomized controlled trials. BMC Cardiovasc Disord 2019;19(1):18.

25. Chen S, Pürerfellner H, Meyer C, et al. Rhythm control for patients with atrial fibrillation complicated with heart failure in the contemporary era of catheter ablation: a stratified pooled analysis of randomized data. Eur Heart J 2020;41(30):2863–73.

26. Aldaas OM, Lupercio F, Darden D, et al. Meta-analysis of the Usefulness of Catheter Ablation of Atrial Fibrillation in Patients With Heart Failure With Preserved Ejection Fraction. Am J Cardiol 2021;142: 66–73.

27. Androulakis E, Sohrabi C, Briasoulis A, et al. Catheter Ablation for Atrial Fibrillation in Patients with Heart Failure with Preserved Ejection Fraction: A Systematic Review and Meta-Analysis. J Clin Med 2022;11(2):288.

28. Marrouche NF, Brachmann J, Andresen D, et al. CASTLE-AF Investigators. Catheter Ablation for Atrial Fibrillation with Heart Failure. N Engl J Med 2018;378(5):417–27.

29. Kuck KH, Merkely B, Zahn R, et al. Catheter Ablation Versus Best Medical Therapy in Patients With Persistent Atrial Fibrillation and Congestive Heart Failure: The Randomized AMICA Trial. Circ Arrhythm Electrophysiol 2019;12(12):e007731.

30. Prabhu S, Taylor AJ, Costello BT, et al. Catheter Ablation Versus Medical Rate Control in Atrial Fibrillation and Systolic Dysfunction: The CAMERA-MRI Study. J Am Coll Cardiol 2017;70(16):1949–61.

31. Di Biase L, Mohanty P, Mohanty S, et al. Ablation Versus Amiodarone for Treatment of Persistent Atrial Fibrillation in Patients With Congestive Heart Failure and an Implanted Device: Results From the AATAC Multicenter Randomized Trial. Circulation 2016; 133(17):1637–44.

32. Zylla MM, Leiner J, Rahm AK, et al. Catheter Ablation of Atrial Fibrillation in Patients With Heart Failure and Preserved Ejection Fraction. Circ Heart Fail 2022;15(9):e009281.

33. Arora S, Jaswaney R, Jani C, et al. Catheter Ablation for Atrial Fibrillation in Patients With Concurrent Heart Failure. Am J Cardiol 2020;137:45–54.

34. Packer DL, Mark DB, Robb RA, et al. CABANA Investigators. Effect of Catheter Ablation vs Antiarrhythmic Drug Therapy on Mortality, Stroke, Bleeding, and Cardiac Arrest Among Patients With Atrial Fibrillation: The CABANA Randomized Clinical Trial. JAMA 2019;321(13):1261–74.

35. Pocock SJ, Stone GW. The Primary Outcome Fails – What Next? N Engl J Med 2016;375:861–70.

36. Packer DL, Piccini JP, Monahan KH, et al. CABANA Investigators. Ablation Versus Drug Therapy for Atrial Fibrillation in Heart Failure: Results From the CABANA Trial. Circulation 2021;143(14):1377–90.

37. Kirchhof P, Camm AJ, Goette A, et al. EAST-AFNET 4 Trial Investigators. Early Rhythm-Control Therapy in Patients with Atrial Fibrillation. N Engl J Med 2020; 383(14):1305–16.

38. Parkash R, Wells GA, Rouleau J, et al. Randomized Ablation-Based Rhythm-Control Versus Rate-Control Trial in Patients With Heart Failure and Atrial Fibrillation: Results from the RAFT-AF trial. Circulation 2022; 145(23):1693–704.

39. Sridhar AR, Yarlagadda V, Parasa S, et al. Cardiac Resynchronization Therapy: US Trends and Disparities in Utilization and Outcomes. Circ Arrhythm Electrophysiol 2016;9(3):e003108.

40. Moss AJ, Hall WJ, Cannom DS, et al. Cardiac-resynchronization therapy for the prevention of heart-failure events. N Engl J Med 2009;361(14):1329–38.

41. Kalscheur MM, Saxon LA, Lee BK, et al. Outcomes of cardiac resynchronization therapy in patients with intermittent atrial fibrillation or atrial flutter in the COMPANION trial. Heart Rhythm 2017;14(6): 858–65.

42. Hoppe UC, Casares JM, Eiskjaer H, et al. Effect of cardiac resynchronization on the incidence of atrial fibrillation in patients with severe heart failure. Circulation 2006;114(1):18–25.

43. Ruwald AC, Kutyifa V, Ruwald MH, et al. The association between biventricular pacing and cardiac resynchronization therapy-defibrillator efficacy when compared with implantable cardioverter defibrillator on outcomes and reverse remodelling. Eur Heart J 2015;36(7):440–8.

44. Gasparini M, Galimberti P, Ceriotti C. The importance of increased percentage of biventricular pacing to improve clinical outcomes in patients receiving cardiac resynchronization therapy. Curr Opin Cardiol 2013 Jan;28(1):50–4. PMID: 23196776.

45. Khan MN, Jaïs P, Cummings J, et al. PABA-CHF Investigators. Pulmonary-vein isolation for atrial fibrillation in patients with heart failure. N Engl J Med 2008; 359(17):1778–85.

46. Brignole M, Pentimalli F, Palmisano P, et al. APAF-CRT Trial Investigators. AV junction ablation and cardiac resynchronization for patients with permanent atrial fibrillation and narrow QRS: the APAF-CRT mortality trial. Eur Heart J 2021;42(46):4731–9. Erratum in: Eur Heart J. 2021 Oct 16;; Erratum in: Eur Heart J. 2021 Dec 08;; PMID: 34453840.

47. Van Gelder IC, Groenveld HF, Crijns HJ, et al. RACE II Investigators. Lenient versus strict rate control in patients with atrial fibrillation. N Engl J Med 2010; 362(15):1363–73.

48. Huang W, Su L, Wu S, et al. Long-term outcomes of His bundle pacing in patients with heart failure with left bundle branch block. Heart 2019;105(2): 137–43.

49. Huang W, Su L, Wu S, et al. A Novel Pacing Strategy With Low and Stable Output: Pacing the Left Bundle Branch Immediately Beyond the Conduction Block. Can J Cardiol 2017;33(12):1736.e1–3.

50. Vijayaraman P, Mathew AJ, Naperkowski A, et al. Conduction system pacing versus conventional pacing in patients undergoing atrioventricular node ablation: Nonrandomized, on-treatment comparison. Heart Rhythm O2 2022;3(4):368–76.

51. Pujol-López M, Jiménez Arjona R, Guasch E, et al. Conduction system pacing vs. biventricular pacing in patients with ventricular dysfunction and AV block. Pacing Clin Electrophysiol 2022;45(9):1115–23.

52. Ivanovski M, Mrak M, Mežnar AZ, et al. Biventricular versus Conduction System Pacing after Atrioventricular Node Ablation in Heart Failure Patients with Atrial Fibrillation. J Cardiovasc Dev Dis 2022; 9(7):209.

Novel Approaches to Sleep Apnea in Heart Failure

Gregory R. Jackson, MD[a],*, Abhinav Singh, MD, MPH[b]

KEYWORDS

- Sleep apnea • Heart failure • Sleep devices • CPAP • OSA • CSA • Cheyne-stokes

KEY POINTS

- Sleep apnea affects ~50% to 75% of patients with heart failure.
- Sleep apnea often goes underrecognized, underdiagnosed, and undertreated in the heart failure population.
- Advanced positive airway pressure algorithms and interfaces allow for improved comfort and adherence.
- Novel therapies such as hypoglossal nerve stimulation, phrenic nerve stimulation, new-generation adaptive servo-ventilation devices, and other developing technologies are emerging as treatment options for sleep apnea.

INTRODUCTION, EPIDEMIOLOGY, AND DEFINITIONS

Sleep apnea is defined as a serious sleep disorder that occurs when breathing is interrupted during sleep. Also referred to as sleep-disordered breathing (SDB), it can be divided into obstructive sleep apnea (OSA) which is caused by a blockage of the airway—usually when soft tissue in the back of the throat collapses during sleep—and central sleep apnea (CSA) caused by intermittent interruption of neural signaling from the respiratory control center leading to cessation of respiratory muscle activity and ventilation and mixed OSA and CSA.

SDB is characterized by apneas (cessation of breathing for >10 seconds) and hypopneas (decreased amplitude of breathing for >10 seconds). SDB is common in heart failure patients and is an independent risk factor for increased mortality. Prevalence rates are between 50% and 75%, rising to 44% to 97% during acute heart failure decompensation.[1] OSA has been associated with an increased risk of death in patients with heart failure independent of confounding factors.[2] Poor cardiovascular outcomes are hypothesized to be due to (1) apneic episodes causing intermittent hypoxemia and increased sympathetic nervous system activity and (2) negative intrathoracic pressures resulting in increased ventricular wall tension and lower stroke volume.

SDB is very common and, even today, remains underdiagnosed in both the general population and heart failure population. The overlap of presenting symptoms with other cardiopulmonary, metabolic, and endocrine disorders likely adds to the delay in diagnosis. It is estimated that in North America, the prevalence of OSA—the most common form of SDB—is 15% to 30% in males and 10% to 15% in females in the general population.[3,4] Global prevalence of OSA is close to one billion adults worldwide.[5] Heart failure remains a major public health problem.[6] Many studies show that about 50% of patients with heart failure, both heart failure with reduced ejection fraction (HFrEF) and heart failure with preserved ejection fraction (HFpEF), have moderate to severe sleep apnea (defined as apnea-hypopnea index [AHI] greater than 15 events per hour).[7–10]

For the purposes of this discussion, we will limit ourselves to the 2 most common forms of SDB seen in patients with heart failure, OSA and

[a] Medical University of South Carolina, Ralph H. Johnson Veterans Affairs Medical Center, Thurmond Gazes Building, 30 Courtenay Drive, BM206, MSC592, Charleston, SC 29425, USA; [b] Indiana Sleep Center, Marian University College of Osteopathic Medicine, 701 East County Line Road Suite 207, Greenwood, IN 46143, USA
* Corresponding author.
E-mail address: jacksogr@musc.edu

Heart Failure Clin 20 (2024) 29–38
https://doi.org/10.1016/j.hfc.2023.05.007
1551-7136/24/Published by Elsevier Inc.

CSA–Cheyne-Stokes breathing (CSA-CSB). Although OSA is much more common than CSA in the general population, patients with heart failure (both with HFpEF and HFrEF) have increased CSA-CSB, and patients with HFrEF are likely to exhibit predominant CSA-CSB.[8,11–13]

DIAGNOSIS AND TESTING

Pathophysiologic mechanisms of central apneas in heart failure are complex. At the core, they involve a delay in transfer of information of CO_2 levels due to prolonged arterial circulation time.[14] Potential causes include dilation of cardiac chambers, reduced cardiac output, and increased pulmonary blood volume. This leads to loop gain instability, which manifests as exaggerated ventilatory response frequently breaching the apneic threshold, leading to the cycles of central apnea-hyperventilation-central apnea, termed Cheyne-Stokes respiration.

Mechanisms leading to obstructive apneas are also multifactorial in heart failure. Central apneas can predispose to airway collapse, especially toward the nadir of the ventilatory cycle as airway dilator muscle tone is low. In addition, there is increased venous congestion in the upper airway, rostral fluid shifts in the supine posture, and obesity—all of which are commonly seen with heart failure—which can increase the risk of obstructive apnea events.

Recurring obstructive and central apneas lead to blood gas turbulence including hypoxia-reoxygenation, hypocapnia-hypercapnia, sleep fragmentation from deeper to lighter states of sleep, and large negative swings in intrathoracic pressure. Physiologically, chronic apnea can lead to oxygen desaturation, decreased arousal, and intrathoracic pressure changes. As a result, there is increased sympathetic activation, endothelial dysfunction, inflammation, oxidative stress, and hypercoagulability. In both heart failure and sleep apnea, endothelial dysfunction manifests with impairments in vasodilatation and decreased availability of nitric oxide, with increases in tumor necrosis factor-α, interleukin-6, and endothelin. These phenomena can negatively affect cardiovascular function, especially in the setting of established coronary artery disease and left ventricular dysfunction.[14] Untreated sleep apnea can result in uncontrolled hypertension, coronary ischemia, myocardial infarction, atrial and ventricular arrhythmias, pulmonary hypertension, right heart failure, left heart failure, polycythemia, stroke, diabetes, arrhythmia, and sudden death.[15]

Excess morbidity, readmissions, and increased mortality are seen in patients with HF and SDB, both OSA and CSA-CSB, compared with those without. The AHI appears to be a strong predictor of mortality, especially in heart failure patients with CSA-CSB[16–19] (Figs. 1 and 2).

Many studies from around the world have demonstrated that treating OSA and CSA reverses the increased sympathetic activity and lowers mortality and readmissions. In 3 of the 5 randomized clinical trials of the continuous positive airway pressure (CPAP) therapy for OSA in patients with HFrEF, significant improvements in ejection fractions of 10%, 5%, and 2% (when compared with the control group) were reported with CPAP use.[20–22] Adherence to the PAP therapy (hours of CPAP use) appeared to be one of the important factors and was proportional to effect size. However, there are other studies that showed no benefit in cardiovascular outcomes and will be discussed later. We feel these neutral outcomes may be in part due to patient selection (excluding severe and sleepy cases) and lower CPAP adherence thresholds in treatment arms. (Sleepy refers to the sleep apneic; diagnosed with moderate to severe OSA, with AHI greater than 15 hours, and are sleepy [typically using a sleepiness questionnaire such as the Epworth

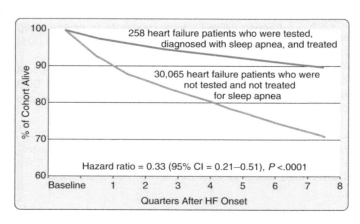

Fig. 1. Medicare beneficiaries who were diagnosed with new heart failure. The 2-year survival of the 258 patients who were tested, diagnosed, and treated for sleep apnea was much better than the survival of the 30,065 patients who were not tested for sleep apnea. The survival was adjusted for age, gender, and Charlson Comorbidity index. (*Adapted from* Javaheri S, Caref EB, Chen E, Tong KB, Abraham WT. Sleep apnea testing and outcomes in a large cohort of Medicare beneficiaries with newly diagnosed heart failure. Am J Respir Crit Care Med. 2011;183(4):539-546.)

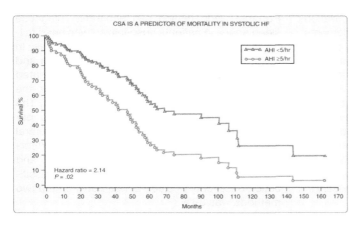

Fig. 2. Probability of survival in patients with systolic heart failure according to the presence or absence of central sleep apnea (CSA). AHI, apnea-hypopnea index. (*From* Javaheri S, Shukla R, Zeigler H, Wexler L. Central sleep apnea, right ventricular dysfunction, and low diastolic blood pressure are predictors of mortality in systolic heart failure. J Am Coll Cardiol. 2007;49(20):2028-2034.)

Sleepiness Scale > 10 out of 24 is deemed excessively sleepy.]; **Fig. 3**)

Who Should We Screen?

Given the broad overlap of sleep apnea and heart failure symptoms such as nonrestorative sleep, daytime sleepiness, fatigue, nocturia, and night time awakening, every patient should be screened for SDB. This can be in the form of a history (related to snoring or unusual breathing pattern at night), questionnaires (STOP-BANG or BERLIN) for

OSA,[23,24] physical examination to include airway anatomy including Mallampati score, jaw adequacy, neck circumference, and body mass index (BMI). Obesity is an important risk factor for the development of OSA. Patients with HFrEF and OSA are heavier, snore habitually, and have higher blood pressures than those with CSA. CSA can be harder to suspect and diagnose than OSA as obesity and snoring—hallmarks of OSA—are often missing. Certain clues such as lower left ventricular ejection fraction (LVEF), nocturnal arrhythmias, and symptomatic heart failure (worse New York Heart

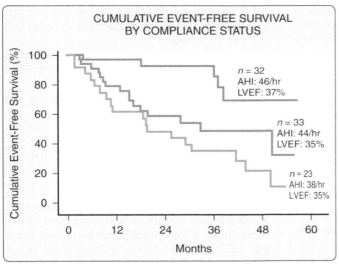

Fig. 3. Probability of hospitalization and mortality in patients with heart failure and obstructive sleep apnea decreases when treated with continuous positive airway pressure (CPAP) and adhere to therapy. AHI, apnea-hypopnea index; HR, hazard ratio; LVEF, left ventricular ejection fraction. (*From* Kasai T, Narui K, Dohi T, et al. Prognosis of patients with heart failure and obstructive sleep apnea treated with continuous positive airway pressure. Chest. 2008;133(3):690-696.)

Association [NYHA] class) and atrial fibrillation should raise suspicion of CSA. As several elements of history rely on a bed partner or a witness, a sleep study is often required. If unable to screen all heart failure patients, those with resistant hypertension, uncontrolled atrial fibrillation, high premature ventricular contraction (PVC) burden, fatigue out of proportion to severity of heart failure, and BMI greater than 35 warrant evaluation. Interestingly, patients with sleep apnea and heart failure are less likely to be sleepy and report daytime fatigue than patients with sleep apnea without heart failure. Therefore, a broader testing strategy may be necessary in this patient population.

Sleep Apnea Testing

Sleep apnea testing can be achieved with a home sleep apnea test or an in-lab polysomnography (PSG). While a home sleep apnea test may have the advantage of lower cost and convenience of testing at home, it is only recommended for a high pretest probability of uncomplicated moderate to severe OSA. It may not detect CSA as accurately and does not offer an opportunity to intervene with PAP. It is important to note that true sleep is not measured, and this often underestimates the true burden of sleep apnea. Lab-based PSG is considered the gold standard and should be considered especially in cases of symptomatic heart failure. Along with measuring true electroencephalogram (EEG) signatures of sleep states, it offers accurate distinction of obstructive and central apneas along with an opportunity to intervene with PAP therapy.

Inpatient Diagnosis and Early Initiation of Treatment

With the advent of the COVID-19 pandemic, there was a major shift in health care in the United States toward telemedicine and virtual health platforms. In addition to staff shortages and decreasing in-person encounters to minimize exposure and spread of disease, there were simplified sleep testing modalities for home-based testing. In addition, at many medical centers, there are delays from time of referral to in-lab sleep testing, delays from test completion to initiation of therapies, and delays in referral to sleep medicine physicians. Home-based testing, in the form of respiratory polygraphy, allows patients the ability to undergo sleep testing in a more peaceful home environment and expedite workup and treatment of SDB.

In addition to home-based testing, there is the opportunity to test and diagnose patients with SDB during the heart failure hospitalization.

Portable sleep testing can accurately diagnose sleep apnea in patients hospitalized with heart failure and allow for early initiation of therapies. In comparing concurrent respiratory polygraph and PSG in hospitalized patients with decompensated heart failure, the correlation coefficient for the overall AHI from the two methods was 0.94. The average difference in AHI was 3.6 events per hour between the two methods. Analysis of central and obstructive AHI values showed strong concordance, with correlation coefficients of 0.98 and 0.91, respectively. Complete agreement in classification of severity of sleep apnea between the two methods was 89%.[25]

In-hospital testing has not only shown accuracy in diagnosis of sleep apnea, with ability to make the diagnosis and initiate therapy sooner, but has also demonstrated the ability to lower heart failure readmissions and lead to lower total cost of care at 6 months following heart failure hospitalization.[26–29] In-hospital testing can be accurately completed following diuresis and decongestion, usually in the last 1 to 2 days of hospitalization before discharge. This was shown by Aurora and colleagues (Portable Sleep Monitoring for Diagnosing Sleep Apnea in Hospitalized Patients with Heart Failure, Chest, 2018 Jul; 154(1)" 91–98).

However, there are a lot of practical limitations which may still limit accurate sleep testing in the hospitalized patients:

- Patients not in their usual sleep environment.
- Diuretics may cause patients to wake up and fragment sleep.
- Patients have increased levels of stress in the hospital, leading to less deep sleep/REM sleep.
- Blood draws and early morning testing can fragment sleep.
- If on supplemental oxygen, cannot typically do portable testing.
- If head of bed (HOB) is elevated, there is reduced accuracy.

Insurance companies may cover this, but it is not frequently done. This is likely a combination of DRG-based limitations and manpower limitations. To run a Type 1 (full in-lab equivalent setup with EEG/electrooculography/chest belts setup) requires additional staffing resources, or Type 3 home sleep test may be less accurate given inability to detect sleep and less-accurate central apnea detection.

TREATMENTS

As goal-directed medical therapy (GDMT) for heart failure is being maximally optimized, the treatment of sleep apnea in heart failure is governed by the predominant phenotype—obstructive or central. For the OSA predominant type, treatment remains largely similar to that for the general population without HF. This is broadly classified into PAP therapy versus non-PAP options.

Non-PAP options include weight loss, posture therapy (avoiding supine posture), exercise,[30] minimizing the use of benzodiazepines, opioids, alcohol, and tobacco[31,32] (simultaneously increases cardiac burden and upper-airway inflammation) and phosphodiesterase inhibitors, such as sildenafil.[33] Mandibular advancement therapies[34] have demonstrated efficacy and do require repeat testing to confirm efficacy. Overall data remain limited for non-PAP options in patients with HF. PAP therapy, often felt to be the most reliable treatment of choice, includes CPAP, auto-PAP (auto titrating algorithms based on event-detection proprietary algorithms relying on airflow resistance), and Bi-level PAP (especially for CPAP noncompliant patients who experience exhalation pressure intolerance). CPAP use in patients with HF improves LVEF, BP, and ventricular systolic volume.[20,21,34] Observational studies have shown improvement in survival in CPAP-compliant patients.[22,26] Implantable hypoglossal nerve stimulators are available for CPAP-intolerant patients with a lower BMI (<32) with moderate to severe OSA (AHI 15–65/h). However, patients with NYHA III-IV symptoms were excluded.

For central predominant type, treatment algorithms are not as straightforward. PAP therapy efficacy and outcomes are not uniform compared with its obstructive counterpart. Nearly half of HF patients with CSA remain unresponsive to CPAP,[35,36] as discussed in more detail below based on trials such as CANPAP, SERVE-HF, and other ongoing trials. For patients with HF and CSA who remain nonresponsive to CPAP after GDMT is optimized, options may be explored as follows.

- Currently ASV-PAP (adaptive servo-ventilation) therapy may be used in patients with CSA and HF with EF greater than 45%. Based on the results of the SERVE-HF trial, there is a recommendation against use in patients for CSA with reduced EF less than 45%, due to 34% increased mortality and cardiovascular death compared with the control group, with no benefit on quality of life or heart failure symptoms.
- Supplemental nocturnal oxygen therapy can help improve CSA, quality of life, desaturations, and increase LVEF (by ~5% compared to 1% in controls).[37,38]

- Theophylline—a centrally acting respiratory stimulant, adenosine competitor—was shown to reduce AHI by 50% and improve arterial oxygen saturations.[39,40] Potential arrhythmogenicity and phosphodiesterase inhibition effects of theophylline should be kept in mind when considering long-term therapy in patients with heart failure.
- Acetazolamide (3 mg/kg) administered 30 minutes before bedtime was shown to reduce central AHI from 57/h (placebo arm) to 34/h. Improvement in oxygen saturations and subjective perception of sleep quality, daytime sleepiness, and fatigue also improved.[41,42] Acetazolamide, being a mild diuretic, may have additional advantage in being able to normalize alkalemia caused by loop diuretics in patients with HF. In one study, pH of 7.43 dropped to 7.37 (in 12 patients with HF in a double-blind crossover study).[42]

Heart Transplant and Left Ventricular Assist Devices

Despite correction of low cardiac output and volume overload following cardiac transplantation, sleep apnea can remain present. In general, CSA is eliminated, suggesting that severe or end-stage heart failure may be causative of CSA. However, more than a third of patients can develop OSA within several months after heart transplant due to weight gain, hypertension, poor quality of life, and perhaps rejection.[43] More recent data show that CSA can be eliminated following left ventricular assist device therapy.[44] As the number of heart failure patients receiving these therapies continues to increase in the United States, further research is warranted in this area (**Fig. 4**).

PAST, PRESENT, AND FUTURE CLINICAL TRIALS

In patients with heart failure, untreated OSA is associated with an increased risk of death.[16] Positive airway pressure therapies have demonstrated mixed results in heart failure patients. In heart failure patients with CSA-CSB randomized to treatment with CPAP, there was a statistically significant improvement in transplant-free survival.[45] In the CANPAP trial, CPAP attenuated CSA, improved nocturnal oxygenation, increased the ejection fraction, lowered norepinephrine levels, and increased the distance walked in 6 minutes. However, CPAP therapy in CSA did not affect survival.[35] In the SERVE-HF trial, treatment with ASV in patients with HFrEF and CSA lead to increased composite risk of death from any cause,

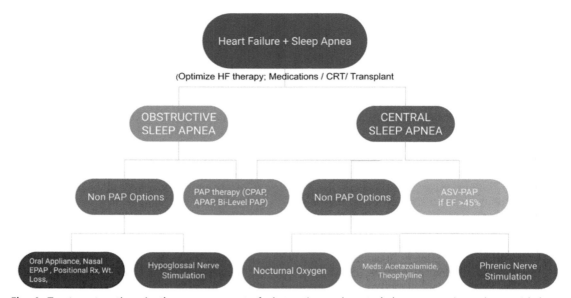

Fig. 4. Treatment options in the management of obstructive and central sleep apnea in patients with heart failure.

a lifesaving cardiovascular intervention, unplanned hospitalization for worsening chronic heart failure, as well as death from any cause, and death from cardiovascular cause.[46] As a result, the use of ASV in patients with HFrEF and CSA may increase mortality and is not advised with a Class III recommendation in the 2017 American College of Cardiology/American Heart Association/Heart Failure Society of America Heart Failure management guidelines.[47] Although the SERVE-HF trial demonstrated 34% increase in cardiovascular mortality in HFrEF patients treated with ASV, it is considered by many that the trial employed older PAP algorithms, had high cross-over rates for a homogenous patient population, used fixed EPAP whereas there is now flexible adaptive EPAP, and the company has since stopped manufacturing the ASV device used in the study. It is felt ASV may still provide benefit to some heart failure patients with sleep apnea. As a result, the ADVENT-HF trial is currently in progress and designed to examine whether advanced ASV and auto-EPAP titration improve cardiovascular outcomes in HFrEF patients with OSA and CSA. Complete data are soon to be released; however, preliminary data show better compliance with ASV than previous trials and no safety concerns to date.[48,49] In addition, the Impact of Low Flow Nocturnal Oxygen Therapy on Hospital Admissions and Mortality in Patients with Heart Failure and Central Sleep Apnea (LOFT-HF) trial is also currently under study and will examine the long-term effects of nocturnal oxygen on the mortality and morbidity of patients with stable HFrEF.[50]

NOVEL TREATMENTS

Obesity is the leading cause of OSA. As many patients with heart failure and sleep apnea suffer from comorbid obesity, attention should be focused on weight loss treatments. Bariatric surgery has also shown to be effective in reducing AHI and quality of life in obese heart failure patients with sleep apnea. More recent data from the INTERAPNEA randomized clinical trial demonstrated that an 8-week interdisciplinary weight loss and lifestyle management intervention were effective in decreasing OSA severity as measured by AHI.[51] Over half of the study participants no longer required CPAP therapy at 6 months after the intervention, and 29.4% experienced a complete remission of OSA at 6 months. The study participants in the weight loss intervention group also experienced greater improvements in body weight and fat mass body composition, lower blood pressure, and improved Sleep Apnea Quality of Life Index. This suggests that intensive nonsurgical weight loss interventions, in addition to new pharmacologic agents with proven cardiovascular benefit such as GLP-1 agonists and SGLT2 inhibitors, can be effective in the treatment of OSA and should be a focus of sleep apnea management.

As trials continue to examine the effect of external PAP device therapies, newer implantable devices for sleep apnea in heart failure patients have emerged in recent years.

Newer noninvasive daytime device-based therapies are also emerging for treatment of OSA. The eXciteOSA device is an FDA-approved, daytime therapy for mild OSA and snoring. The device is intended for use for 20 minutes daily, while awake, and uses neuromuscular electrical stimulation to strengthen tongue muscles which get weak and obstruct the airway during sleep, resulting in OSA. In early efficacy trials of the device, 90% of the study population experienced some reduction in objective snoring with a mean reduction of 41%, as well as reduction in bed partner-reported snoring, improved bed partner sleep quality, and improved patient daytime somnolence.[52] The device mouthpiece requires replacement every 90 days.

The Inspire upper airway stimulation (UAS) device (Inspire Medical Systems), a hypoglossal nerve stimulator, has emerged as an implantable device for treatment of moderate to severe OSA. This novel device consists of a small impulse generator implanted beneath the clavicle, a breathing sensor placed between the intercostal and external muscles, and a stimulation lead attached to the branch of the hypoglossal nerve that controls tongue protrusion. When the sensing lead detects inspiration, the impulse generator sends a signal via the stimulation lead to the hypoglossal nerve, resulting in slight forward displacement of the stiffened tongue and reduction in airway obstruction. It was initially studied in the Stimulation Therapy for Apnea Reduction (STAR) trial and demonstrated a 68% reduction in AHI, 70% reduction in oxygen desaturation index, and improvement in functional outcomes of sleep questionnaire quality of life metrics and Epworth Sleepiness Scale.[53] The Inspire device is used for adults who have failed or cannot tolerate PAP treatments (CPAP, Bi-level PAP) and do not have complete airway collapse during inspiration. The impulse generator is similar in size to that of a cardiac pacemaker, and the newer-generation device is MRI-compatible. Although patients with NYHA class III and IV heart failure were excluded from this trial, subsequent studies demonstrated that simultaneous use of a hypoglossal nerve UAS device is safe, effective, and without device-device interactions when used in patients with cardiac implantable electronic devices.[41] However, this device has not been well studied in patients with heart failure, and the impact on cardiovascular outcomes is unknown (**Fig. 5**).

The Genio hypoglossal neurostimulator (Nyxoah S.A.) is currently pursuing FDA approval. This device places stimulator electrodes bilaterally in contact with both branches of the hypoglossal nerve, with a single incision under the chin and a leadless and battery-free platform. The neurostimulator triggers the tongue muscles to maintain an open airway during sleep. The system requires an external activation chip, which is connected to a

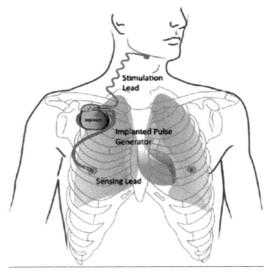

Fig. 5. Inspire device, hypoglossal nerve stimulator. (*From* Van de Heyning PH, Badr MS, Baskin JZ, et al. Implanted upper airway stimulation device for obstructive sleep apnea. Laryngoscope. 2012;122(7):1626-1633.)

disposable patch and replaced every night. In 2020, the FDA approved an Investigational Device Exemption (IDE) to begin the Dual-sided Hypoglossal neRvE stimulAtion for the treatMent of Obstructive Sleep Apnea (DREAM) study.[42] The company is also developing new technologies that will treat SDB through stimulation of the ansa cervicalis, the efferent fiber of the glossopharyngeal nerve or nerves that innervate the palatoglossus and/or the palatopharyngeal muscle.

Another UAS device, the aura6000 (LivaNova), is currently approved in Europe and awaiting FDA approval. The device provides mild stimulation pulses via a lead to the hypoglossal nerve from a rechargeable, implantable pulse generator. In 2021, LivaNova was granted FDA IDE to initiate the Treating Obstructive Sleep Apnea using Targeted Hypoglossal Neurostimulation (OSPREY) clinical study. The OSPREY study will seek to demonstrate safety and effectiveness of the aura6000 system in patients with moderate to severe OSA.

The remedē device (Zoll Medical Corporation) is an implantable diaphragmatic stimulator for the treatment of CSA. With this device, a stimulation lead is placed in the left pericardiophrenic or right brachiocephalic vein to stimulate the phrenic nerve, while the sensing lead is placed in a thoracic vein, such as the azygos vein, to sense respiration via thoracic impedance. The remedē System Therapy (reST) study is ongoing, as a nonrandomized postmarket registry to collect clinical data on the safety and effectiveness of the remedē

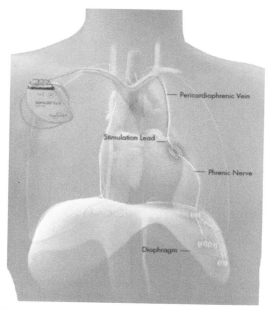

Fig. 6. Remedē device demonstrating right-sided generator with left-sided stimulation lead. (Image reproduced with permission from ZOLL Medical.)

system in real-world study of patients with moderate to severe CSA and AHI greater than 15 events/h. The trial will include heart failure patients and will provide insight into device-based therapies for patients with HFrEF and CSA. Data presented at CHEST and HFSA annual meetings in 2020 demonstrated improvement in sleep, breathing, and quality of life, with a 96% reduction in central apneas[50] (**Fig. 6**).

SUMMARY

Given the negative impact of OSA and CSA on patients with heart failure, we urge all clinicians to screen as early as possible. New technology continues to emerge in both the diagnosis and management of sleep apnea in heart failure patients. This includes home sleep tests, in-hospital sleep testing, telemedicine, remote monitoring and cloud-based monitoring platforms, newer weight loss medications, and both invasive and noninvasive device-based therapies. PAP therapies are a noninvasive, safe, cost-effective, and reliable way to treat OSA with the added advantage of easy remote monitoring. With more than 160 interfaces, humidity, pressure relief during exhalation, auto PAP algorithms, and modalities such as Bi-level PAP available, new device options offer patients increased comfort and improved adherence to therapies. For patients who have continued difficulty with PAP therapy or claustrophobia, PAP desensitization can help improve compliance.

Non-PAP options include weight loss, posture therapy, oral appliance therapy, nasal EPAP therapy, and hypoglossal nerve stimulation therapy for OSA. Non-PAP options for CSA exist and include nocturnal oxygen, medications, and newer implantable devices such as phrenic nerve stimulators which make for increased choices. Including sleep medicine clinicians in multidisciplinary heart failure clinics may allow for more comprehensive patient education, streamlined treatment modality choices, and overall improved outcomes.

Sleep is at the heart of the matter, and a very important matter for the heart.

CLINICS CARE POINTS

Diagnosis

Testing—home-based study versus in-lab testing

In-lab testing:

- Remains gold standard, especially in symptomatic heart failure patients.

Home-based test disadvantages:

- *True sleep is not captured and PAP intervention not possible (especially for those who have* tried and failed in the past).
- Central apneas/CSR cannot be accurately estimated on home testing.
- Underestimates overall severity.
- Cardiac rhythms not characterized.

Treatments

- Non-PAP therapies (for OSA only)
  - Weight loss
  - Posture therapies
  - Nasal EPAP therapies
  - Oral appliance therapies
  - Hypoglossal nerve stimulation
  - Surgical therapies ENT based—not frequently performed (omitted based on scope of this article)
  - Bariatric surgery
- PAP therapies
  - CPAP, APAP (OSA-predominant pathology)
  - Bi-Level PAP, ± backup rate (for central events)
  - Servo ventilation therapies for CSA/CSR (EF >45%)
  - Supplemental oxygen therapy

DISCLOSURE

The authors have no disclosures, commercial or financial conflicts of interest related to the writing of this manuscript.

REFERENCES

1. Cowie MR, Linz D, Redline S, et al. Sleep Disordered Breathing and Cardiovascular Disease: JACC State-of-the-Art Review. J Am Coll Cardiol 2021;78(6): 608–24.
2. Wang H, Parker JD, Newton GE, et al. Influence of Obstructive Sleep Apnea on Mortality in Patients With Heart Failure. J Am Coll Cardiol 2007;49(15):1625–31.
3. Young T, Palta M, Dempsey J, et al. Burden of sleep apnea: rationale, design, and major findings of the Wisconsin Sleep Cohort study. Wis Med J 2009;108(5):246.
4. Peppard PE, Young T, Barnet JH, et al. Increased prevalence of sleep-disordered breathing in adults. Am J Epidemiol 2013;177(9):1006.
5. Benjafield AV, Ayas NT, Eastwood PR, et al. Estimation of the global prevalence and burden of obstructive sleep apnoea: a literature-based analysis. Lancet Respir Med 2019;7(8):687.
6. Virani SS, Alonso A, Benjamin EJ, et al. Heart Disease and Stroke Statistics-2020 Update: A Report from the American Heart Association. Circulation 2020;141(9):e139–596.
7. Javaheri S, Parker TJ, Liming JD, et al. Sleep apnea in 81 ambulatory male patients with stable heart failure. Types and their prevalences, consequences, and presentations. Circulation 1998;97:2154.
8. Corrà U, Pistono M, Mezzani A, et al. Sleep and exertional periodic breathing in chronic heart failure: prognostic importance and interdependence. Circulation 2006;113(1):44.
9. Javaheri S, Parker TJ, Wexler L, et al. Occult sleep-disordered breathing in stable congestive heart failure. Ann Intern Med 1995;122:487.
10. Sin DD, Fitzgerald F, Parker JD, et al. Risk factors for central and obstructive sleep apnea in 450 men and women with congestive heart failure. Am J Respir Crit Care Med 1999;160:1101.
11. Javaheri S, Barbe F, Campos-Rodriguez F, et al. Sleep Apnea: Types, Mechanisms, and Clinical Cardiovascular Consequences. J Am Coll Cardiol 2017; 69(7):841–58.
12. Javaheri S, Brown LK, Abraham WT, et al. Apneas of Heart Failure and Phenotype-Guided Treatments: Part One: OSA. Chest 2020;157(2):394.
13. Bucca CB, Brussino L, Battisti A, et al. Diuretics in obstructive sleep apnea with diastolic heart failure. Chest 2007;132(2):440.
14. Kryger MH, Roth T, Goldstein CA. Principles and Practice of sleep medicine. 7th edition. Heart Failure; 2022. Chapter 149.
15. Sánchez-de-la-Torre M, Campos-Rodriguez F, Barbé F. Obstructive sleep apnoea and cardiovascular disease. Lancet: Respiratory Medicine, March 2013;1(1):61–72.
16. Wang H, Parker JD, Newton GE, et al. Influence of obstructive sleep apnea on mortality in patients with heart failure. J Am Coll Cardiol 2007;49(15):1625–31.
17. Lanfranchi PA, Braghiroli A, Bosimini E, et al. Prognostic value of nocturnal Cheyne-Stokes respiration in chronic heart failure. Circulation 1999;99(11): 1435–40.
18. Dark DS, Pingleton SK, Kerby GR, et al. Breathing pattern abnormalities and arterial oxygen desaturation during sleep in the congestive heart failure syndrome. Improvement following medical therapy. Chest 1987;91(6):833–6.
19. Findley LJ, Zwillich CW, Ancoli-Israel S, et al. Cheyne-Stokes breathing during sleep in patients with left ventricular heart failure. South Med J 1985;78(1):11–5.
20. Egea CJ, Aizpuru F, Pinto JA, et al. Cardiac function after CPAP therapy in patients with chronic heart failure and sleep apnea: a multicenter study. Sleep Med 2008;9(6):660–6.
21. Kaneko Y, Floras JS, Usui K, et al. Cardiovascular effects of continuous positive airway pressure in patients with heart failure and obstructive sleep apnea. N Engl J Med 2003;348(13):1233–41.
22. Mansfield R, Gollogly NC, Kaye DM, et al. Controlled trial of continuous positive airway pressure in obstructive sleep apnea and heart failure. Am J Respir Crit Care Med 2004;169(3):361–6.
23. Chung F, Yegneswaran B, Liao P, et al. STOP Questionnaire: A Tool to Screen Patients for Obstructive Sleep Apnea. Anesthesiology 2008; 108(5):812–21.
24. Netzer NC, Stoohs RA, Netzer CM, et al. Using the Berlin Questionnaire to identify patients at risk for the sleep apnea syndrome. Ann Intern Med 1999; 131:485–91.
25. Aurora RN, Patil SP, Punjabi NM. Portable Sleep Monitoring for Diagnosing Sleep Apnea in Hospitalized Patients With Heart Failure. Chest 2018;154(1):91–8.
26. Javaheri S, Caref EB, Chen E, et al. Sleep apnea testing and outcomes in a large cohort of Medicare beneficiaries with newly diagnosed heart failure. Am J Respir Crit Care Med 2011;183(4):539–46.
27. Khayat RN, Javaheri S, Porter K, et al. In-Hospital Management of Sleep Apnea During Heart Failure Hospitalization: A Randomized Controlled Trial. J Cardiac Fail 2020;26:705–12.
28. Patel N, Porter K, Englert J, et al. Impact of Central Sleep Apnea on the Cost of Heart Failure Readmissions. J Card Fail 2020;26(10S):S116.
29. Kauta SR, Keenan BT, Goldberg L, et al. Diagnosis and Treatment of Sleep Disordered Breathing in Hospitalized Cardiac Patients: A Reduction

in 30-Day Hospital Readmission Rates. J Clin Sleep Med 2014;10(10):1051–9.

30. Iftikhar I.H., Kline C.E., Youngstedt S.D., Effects of Exercise Training on Sleep Apnea: A Meta-analysis, Lung, 192 (1), 2014, 175–184.

31. Pataka A, Kotoulas S, Kalamaras G, et al. Does Smoking Affect OSA? What about Smoking Cessation? J Clin Med 2022;11(17):5164.

32. Javaheri S, Shukla R, Wexler L. Association of smoking, sleep apnea, and plasma alkalosis with nocturnal ventricular arrhythmias in men with systolic heart failure. Chest 2012;141(6):1449–56.

33. Roizenblatt S, Guilleminault C, Poyares D, et al. A double-blind, placebo-controlled, crossover study of sildenafil in obstructive sleep apnea. Arch Intern Med 2006;166(16):1763–7.

34. Eskafi M, Ekberg E, Cline C, et al. Use of a mandibular advancement device in patients with congestive heart failure and sleep apnoea. Gerodontology 2004;21(2):100–7.

35. Bradley TD, Logan AG, Kimoff RJ, et al. Continuous positive airway pressure for central sleep apnea and heart failure. N Engl J Med 2005;353(19):2025–33.

36. Javaheri S. Effects of continuous positive airway pressure on sleep apnea and ventricular irritability in patients with heart failure. Circulation 2000;101(4):392–7.

37. Sasayama S, Izumi T, Seino Y, et al, CHF-HOT Study Group. Effects of nocturnal oxygen therapy on outcome measures in patients with chronic heart failure and cheyne-Stokes respiration. Circ J 2006;70(1):1–7.

38. Toyama T, Seki R, Kasama S, et al. Effectiveness of nocturnal home oxygen therapy to improve exercise capacity, cardiac function and cardiac sympathetic nerve activity in patients with chronic heart failure and central sleep apnea. Circ J 2009;73(2):299–304.

39. Hu K, Li Q, Yang J, et al. The effect of theophylline on sleep-disordered breathing in patients with stable chronic congestive heart failure. Chin Med J (Engl) 2003;116(11):1711–6.

40. Javaheri S, Parker TJ, Wexler L, et al. Effect of theophylline on sleep-disordered breathing in heart failure. N Engl J Med 1996;335(8):562–7.

41. Parikh V, Thaler E, Kato M, et al. Early feasibility of hypoglossal nerve upper airway stimulator in patients with cardiac implantable electronic devices and continuous positive airway pressure-intolerant severe obstructive sleep apnea. Heart Rhythm 2018;15(8):1165–70.

42. Dual-sided Hypoglossal neRvE stimulAtion for the treatMent of Obstructive Sleep Apnea (DREAM). Available at: https://clinicaltrials.gov/ct2/show/NCT03868618. Accessed April 16, 2023.

43. Javaheri S, Abraham W, Brown C, et al. Prevalence of obstructive sleep apnea and periodic limb movement in 45 subjects with heart transplantation. Eur Heart J 2004;25:260–6.

44. Durland JN, Hoyland F, Epps J, et al. Left ventricular assist device (LVAD) resolving central sleep apnea. Am Soc Artif Intern Organs J 2022;68(Supplement 2):115.

45. Sin DD, Logan AG, Fitzgerald FS, et al. Effects of Continuous Positive Airway Pressure on Cardiovascular Outcomes in Heart Failure Patients With and Without Cheyne-Stokes Respiration. Circulation 2000;102(1):61–6.

46. Cowie M.R., Woehrle H., Wegscheider K., et al., Adaptive Servo-Ventilation for Central Sleep Apnea in Systolic Heart Failure, NEJM Sept, 373 (12), 2015, 1095–1105.

47. Yancy C.W., Jessup M., Bozkurt B., et al., 2017 ACC/AHA/HFSA Focused Update of the 2013 ACCF/AHA Guideline for the Management of Heart Failure: A Report of the American College of Cardiology/American Heart Association Task Force on Clinical Practice Guidelines and the Heart Failure Society of America, Circulation, 136 (6), 2017, e137–e161.

48. Perger E, Lyons OD, Inami T, et al. for the ADVENT-HF Investigators. Predictors of 1-year compliance with adaptive servoventilation in patients with heart failure and sleep disordered breathing: preliminary data from the ADVENT-HF trial. Eur Respir J 2019; 53:1801626.

49. Javaheri S, Schwartz A, Abraham W, et al. Effects of Transvenous Phrenic Nerve Stimulation on Central Sleep Apnea and Sleep Architecture: The 5 Year Analysis. Chest 2020;158(4):A2412–3.

50. The Impact of Low Flow Nocturnal Oxygen Therapy on Hospital Admissions and Mortality in Patients With Heart Failure and Central Sleep Apnea. LOFT-HF trial Available at: https://clinicaltrials.gov/ct2/show/NCT03745898. Accessed April 16, 2023.

51. Carneiro-Barrera A, Amaro-Gahete FJ, Guillén-Riquelme A, et al. Effect of an Interdisciplinary Weight Loss and Lifestyle Intervention on Obstructive Sleep Apnea Severity: The INTERAPNEA Randomized Clinical Trial. JAMA Netw Open 2022;5(4):e228212.

52. Baptista PM, Martinez Ruiz de Apodaca P, Carrasco M, et al. Daytime neuromuscular electrical therapy of tongue muscles in improving snoring in individuals with primary snoring and mild obstructive sleep apnea. J Clin Med 2021;10(9):1–11.

53. Strollo PJ Jr, Soose RJ, Maurer JT, et al, STAR Trial Group. Upper-airway stimulation for obstructive sleep apnea. N Engl J Med 2014;370:139–49.

Baroreflex Activation Therapy in Patients with Heart Failure with a Reduced Ejection Fraction

Jean M. Ruddy, MD[a,b,*], Anne Kroman, DO, PhD[b,c], Catalin F. Baicu, PhD[b,c], Michael R. Zile, MD[b,c]

KEYWORDS

- Heart failure • Autonomic nervous system • Baroreflex • Quality of life • Exercise capacity
- Functional status

KEY POINTS

- Baroreflex activation therapy (BAT) is delivered using surgical placement of an extravascular lead that has been shown to be safe with a major adverse neurological or cardiovascular system or procedure-related event free rate of 97%.
- BAT significantly improved patient centered symptomatic outcomes, increasing exercise capacity, improving quality of life, decreasing n-terminal pro B-type natriuretic peptide, and improving functional class.
- BAT mechanism of action includes increased baroreflex sensitivity, increased parasympathetic signaling and decreased sympathetic signaling.

INTRODUCTION

Heart failure (HF) with a reduced ejection fraction (HFrEF) is characterized by the presence of significant autonomic nervous system (ANS) dysfunction.[1–4] Autonomic dysfunction is a pivotal factor in the pathophysiology of the HF syndrome and likely contributes to the residual risk of increased morbidity and mortality that remains even with successful application of guideline-directed management (GDMT).[5–7] Despite HF therapy with all components of GDMT, significant autonomic dysfunction remains and constitutes a critical unmet need and a tangible target for the development of novel HFrEF therapy. Carotid baroreflex activation therapy (BAT) was developed, and recent studies have shown that BAT can modulate and restore the imbalance in cardiac autonomic function present in patients with HFrEF.[8,9] The premarket phase of the a Randomized, Controlled Trial of Baroreflex Activation Therapy in Patients with Heart Failure and Reduced Ejection Fraction (BeAT-HF Trial; ClinicalTrial.gov Identifier: NCT02627196) demonstrated that treatment with BAT for 6 months was safe and significantly improved patient-centered symptomatic outcomes by increasing exercise capacity, improving quality of life (QoL), decrease in n-terminal pro B-type natriuretic peptide (NT-proBNP), and improve functional class.[10] On the basis of these data, BAT was approved by the FDA for the improvement of symptoms of HF for patients who remain symptomatic despite treatment with GDMT, are New York Heart Association (NYHA)

[a] Division of Vascular Surgery, Department of Surgery, Medical University of South Carolina, 30 Courtenay Drive, Charleston, SC 29425, USA; [b] Ralph H Johnson Department of Veterans Affairs Health Care System, 109 Bee Street, Charleston, SC 29401, USA; [c] Division of Cardiology, Department of Medicine, Medical University of South Carolina, 30 Courtenay Drive, Charleston, SC 29425, USA
* Corresponding author. Division of Vascular Surgery, Department of Surgery, Medical University of South Carolina, Thurmond/Gazes, Room 654, 30 Courtenay Drive, Charleston, SC 29425.
E-mail address: ruddy@musc.edu

Heart Failure Clin 20 (2024) 39–50
https://doi.org/10.1016/j.hfc.2023.05.008
1551-7136/24/© 2023 Elsevier Inc. All rights reserved.

Class III or Class II (with a recent history of Class III), have a left ventricular ejection fraction (LVEF) ≤ 35%, an NT-proBNP less than 1600 pg/mL and excluding patients indicated for cardiac resynchronization therapy (CRT) according to the AHA/ACC/ESC guidelines.[5–7] In addition to determine whether BAT has an acceptable long-term safety profile, can improve patient-centered symptomatic outcomes that are durable over time and sustainable in effect, and alter mortality and morbidity will be examined in the post-market phase of BeAT-HF which is scheduled to be completed in 2023.

Autonomic Nervous System Imbalance in Chronic Heart Failure

From a therapeutic viewpoint, cardiologists treating chronic HF largely focus on efferent ANS signaling that modify parasympathetic and sympathetic output (**Fig. 1**A).[1–4] It has been well established in basic, translational, and clinical studies that chronic HF, particularly HFrEF, is characterized by increased sympathetic activity and decreased parasympathetic activity. However, what has become increasingly clear over the past two decades is the importance of alterations in afferent signaling, in particular carotid artery baroreceptor signaling and the integral role baroreceptor signaling plays in maintaining ANS homeostasis (**Fig. 1**B). A number of clinical measurement techniques that quantify baroreflex sensitivity (BRS) have shown that BRS is significantly decreased in HFrEF and these changes in BRS effect the prognosis and symptom status of patients with HFrEF. BRS assessed by blood pressure (BP) response to external applied carotid pressure (**Fig. 2**A), changes in R–R intervals (measured in milliseconds) in response to beat-to-beat changes in BP (measured in mm Hg) induced by intravenous (IV) phenylephrine (**Fig. 2**B), changes in the relationship between muscle sympathetic nerve traffic bursts versus diastolic BP and a number of other measures have all been shown to be abnormal in patients with HFrEF. In addition, the extent to which BRS is reduced is associated with worsening symptom status, decreased survival, and increased rates of HF hospitalization (see **Fig. 2**B–D). Modification of these HFrEF-related abnormalities in autonomic function constitute a critical unmet need and a tangible target for the development of novel HFrEF therapy; this was the goal in development of BAT.

Baroreflex Activation Therapy Mechanism of Action

The 2022 Guidelines described 4 pillars of medical therapy (ACE-I/ARB/ARNI, MRA, β-blockade, SGLT2-i) and 2 device pillars of device therapy (CRT, implantable cardioverter-defibrillator [ICD]) for patients with HFrEF.[7] The underlying *mechanisms of action* by which these Class I-indicated therapies effect a reduction in morbidity and mortality have not been precisely defined in clinical studies of patients with HFrEF. For many, sophisticated hypotheses have been proposed but causal relationships have not been completed tested in human studies. By contrast, the clinical evidence that supports the development of efficacy and safety of BAT in patients with HFrEF has undergone studies in clinically relevant animal models of HFrEF and in patients with HFrEF (**Fig. 3**).

Tonically active arterial baroreceptors form a branching network in the adventitial–medial layers of the carotid sinus and the aortic arch walls. Under normal physiologic conditions, stretch signals due to increases in BP escalate the rate of impulse firing, promote stimulation of the nucleus tractus solitarius, lead to an overall reduction in the sympathetic signaling and increase in parasympathetic signaling from the brain to the heart and other organ systems. Alternatively, reduced BP can decrease nerve firing frequency, reduce

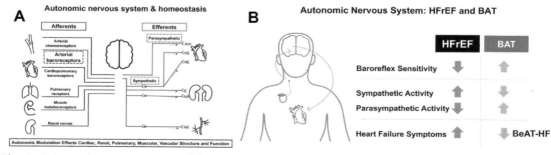

Fig. 1. Autonomic nervous system. (*A*) Homeostatic regulation. (*B*) Autonomic nervous system in patients with HFrEF and the effects of BAT. E, epinephrine; NE, norepinephrine. (From Floras JS. Sympathetic nervous system activation in human heart failure: clinical implications of an updated model. J Am Coll Cardiol. 2009;54(5):375-385.)

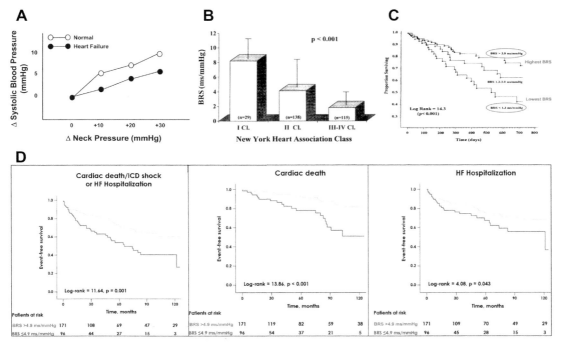

Fig. 2. Relationship between BRS and the severity and prognosis in patients with HFrEF. (*A*) Baroreceptor sensitivity is reduced in HFrEF. (*B*) The extent to which baroreceptor sensitivity is reduced in HFrEF is associated with the severity of symptoms as judged by the NYHA classification. (*C*) The extent to which baroreceptor sensitivity is reduced in HFrEF predicts survival. (*D*) The extent to which baroreceptor sensitivity is reduced in heart failure with a reduced ejection fraction (HFrEF) predicts cardiac death, ICD shocks, or HF hospitalizations. (*From* [*A*] Creager MA, Creager SJ. Arterial baroreflex regulation of blood pressure in patients with congestive heart failure. J Am Coll Cardiol. 1994;23(2):401-405.; [*B*] Mortara A, La Rovere MT, Pinna GD, et al. Arterial baroreflex modulation of heart rate in chronic heart failure: clinical and hemodynamic correlates and prognostic implications. *Circulation*. 1997;96(10):3450-3458.; *Adapted from* [*C*] *From* Mortara A, La Rovere MT, Pinna GD, et al. Arterial baroreflex modulation of heart rate in chronic heart failure: clinical and hemodynamic correlates and prognostic implications. Circulation. 1997;96(10):3450-3458. [*D*] *From* Giannoni A, Gentile F, Buoncristiani F, et al. Chemoreflex and Baroreflex Sensitivity Hold a Strong Prognostic Value in Chronic Heart Failure. JACC Heart Fail. 2022;10(9):662-676.)

nucleus tractus solitarius stimulation, and result in an overall increase of sympathetic signaling and decrease in parasympathetic signaling. Central baroreceptor signals of afferent excitatory pulses to the brain are integrated into a balanced efferent outflow to the heart as well as skeletal muscle, kidney, cardiac mechanoreceptors, and chemoreceptors, which modulate both vagal and sympathetic signaling. These same increased afferent signals and balanced efferent signals are created by electrical stimulation of the carotid baroreceptor (BAT) thus defining a clear mechanism of

Fig. 3. Clinical evidence supporting the development and application of baroreceptor activation therapy in the treatment of HFrEF. Phases I, II, and III are outlined.

Clinical Evidence Development in Heart Failure

	Phase I: BAT in HF 1st Enrollment 12/2011	Phase II: HOPE4HF 1st Enrollment 5/2012	Phase III: BeAT-HF 1st Enrollment 4/2016
Objective	• Assess safety • Demonstrate mechanism of action with GDMT	• Assess safety and Effectiveness	• Demonstrate safety and effectiveness
Study Subjects	• Single Center Studies	• n = 146	• n = 323
Outcomes	• BAT Therapy is safe • Mechanism of action demonstrated through muscle sympathetic nerve activity & HR variability	• BAT Therapy is safe and effective in heart failure • CE Mark Approval	• BAT Therapy is a safe, effective solution for heart failure patients • FDA Approval 8/16/19

action and supporting a strong rationale for the use of BAT in HFrEF.

Animal models of chronic HFrEF provided early indications that BAT was feasible and effective.[11,12] More specifically, in pacing-induced HFrEF, continuous bilateral BAT (50–100 Hz, 0.5–1 msec[2], 2.5–7.5 V) performed using the Rheos system (CVRx, Inc., Minneapolis, MN, USA) had no effect on arterial BP, resting heart rate, or left ventricular pressure, but led to improved survival and suppressed neurohormonal activation.[11] Subsequently, a coronary microembolization-induced HFrEF model employed chronic bilateral BAT using the same system and demonstrated reduced plasma norepinephrine, improved LV function, and favorable LV remodeling (reduced interstitial fibrosis and cardiomyocyte hypertrophy).[12] With these encouraging physiologic and pathologic results, transition to human studies was indicated.

Phase I clinical studies were performed to demonstrate the BAT mechanism of action in patients with HFrEF. During early investigations in patients with resistant hypertension, investigators recognized that unilateral carotid artery stimulator had a more favorable risk profile without sacrificing efficacy, particularly with a right-sided implant.[13,14] A first-in-man, single-center study was initiated utilizing right-sided surgical implantation of a next-generation device, Barostim *neo* system (CVRx Inc., Minneapolis, MN, USA).[8] This approach allowed for confirmation of electrode contact with the carotid sinus as demonstrated by acute stimulation resulting in a BP and heart rate (HR) reduction. The study included 11 patients with advanced HF (67 ± 9 years, all in NYHA Class III, LVEF 31 ± 7%, 46% with chronic renal disease, optimized on goal-directed medical therapy (GDMT) with greater than 90% ACE-I/ARB, β-blocker, mineralocorticoid receptor antagonist [MRA] use, and ineligible for CRT).[8] Following 6 months of BAT, BRS was increased (**Fig. 4**A), muscle sympathetic nerve activity, a reflection of sympathetic signaling, was reduced (**Fig. 4**B). Additional studies in patients with HFrEF demonstrated that BAT reduced sympathetic signaling as evidenced by a reduction in the low frequency component of heart rate variability (HRV) and the parasympathetic signaling was increased as evidenced by an increase in the high-frequency component of HRV (**Fig. 4**C).

Baroreflex Activation Therapy Safety and Effectiveness

The efficacy and safety of BAT was first examined in a Phase II (HOPE4HF), proof of concept, randomized, controlled trial that enrolled 140 patients with NYHA Class III HFrEF, LVEF ≤ 35%, randomized 1:1 to receive GDMT alone (control group) or GDMT plus BAT (BAT group) using the CVRx Barostim Neo System[15] (see **Fig. 3**). In this study, 32% of participants had CRT. The primary efficacy endpoints included NYHA functional Class, QoL score using the Minnesota Living with Heart Failure Questionnaire (MLWHFQ), exercise capacity, using the 6 minute hall walk distance (6MHW), and NT-proBNP, all of which were improved in the BAT group.[15] There was a trend toward fewer in-hospital days for HF exacerbation in BAT group. The beneficial effects of BAT were more pronounced among patients without CRT, potentially attributable to the role that CRT serves in raising cardiac output to reduce abnormal afferent sympathetic signaling, thereby blunting the sympatho-vagal imbalance and limiting the benefits of BAT.[16]

A pivotal Phase III study was then conducted (BeAT-HF, baroreflex activation therapy for heart failure) as the first trial to engage the FDA Breakthrough Devices Program with a complex, interactive and adaptive design (see **Fig. 3**).[17] Baroreflex activation therapy for heart failure was a prospective, multicenter, randomized, 2-arm, parallel-group, open-label with blinded evaluation trial. Subjects were randomized into 2 groups: BAT plus optimal medical management (BAT group) or optimal medical management alone (control group). There were 103 US sites and 5 centers in the United Kingdom. Baroreflex activation therapy for heart failure enrolled patients NYHA Class III or Class II (with a recent history of Class III), LVEF ≤ 35% with a 6MHW 150 to 400 m, with either a previous HF hospitalization or NT-proBNP greater than 400, stable optimal medical management ≥ 4 weeks, no class I indication for CRT and NT-proBNP less than 1600 pg/mL[10] (**Tables 1** and **2**). Participation in the Breakthrough Devices Program facilitated collaboration with the FDA and enabled the BeAT-HF study to be divided into two phases: pre-market-phase and post-market phase.[17] The unique structure of BeAT-HF-enabled preliminary analysis of the early subjects enrolled without NT-proBNP level limitations, showing a lower efficacy of BAT among patients with NT-proBNP greater than 1600 pg/mL, therefore the "intended for use" population was then defined.[8] In the completed pre-market phase, the BAT group demonstrated significant improvement in each of the primary efficacy endpoints (6MHW, QoL, NYHA class, and, NT-proBNP levels; **Fig. 5**), and the freedom from major adverse neurological or cardiovascular events approached 97%.[8]

BAT significantly improved patient-centered symptomatic endpoints (see **Fig. 5**).

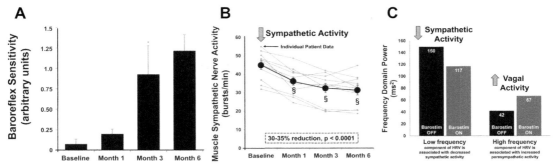

Fig. 4. Effects of baroreflex activation therapy on BRS and sympathetic and parasympathetic signaling, para signaling. (*A*) BAT increases baroreflex sensitivity. (*B*) BAT decreases sympathetic tone. (*C*) Effect of BAT in HFrEF on sympatho-vagal balance. ([*A*] *From* Gronda E, Seravalle G, Brambilla G, et al. Chronic baroreflex activation effects on sympathetic nerve traffic, baroreflex function, and cardiac haemodynamics in heart failure: a proof-of-concept study. Eur J Heart Fail. 2014;16(9):977-983.; *Adapted from* [*B*] *From* Gronda E, Seravalle G, Brambilla G, et al. Chronic baroreflex activation effects on sympathetic nerve traffic, baroreflex function, and cardiac haemodynamics in heart failure: a proof-of-concept study. Eur J Heart Fail. 2014;16(9):977-983; [*C*] *From* Wustmann K, Kucera JP, Scheffers I, et al. Effects of chronic baroreceptor stimulation on the autonomic cardiovascular regulation in patients with drug-resistant arterial hypertension. Hypertension. 2009;54(3):530-536.)

QoL: Assessed using the MLWHFQ, comparing baseline values to those 6 months after randomization demonstrated that compared to control, BAT improved QoL by 14 points (a decrease in score indicated improvement), *P* < .001. A clinically meaningful improvement is considered 5 points or greater. These data favorably compared (and in fact are twice as large) as the changes seen with CRT.

Exercise capacity: Assessed using the 6MHWD improved in the BAT versus control group 6 months after randomization by 60 m, *P* < .001. A clinically meaningful improvement is considered 25 m or greater. These data favorably compared (and in fact are twice as large) as the changes seen with CRT. *Functional status:* Assessed by the NYHA functional class demonstrated that the percentage

Table 1
Baroreflex activation therapy for heart failure baseline demographics for pre-market phase

Variables	BAT (n = 130)	Control (n = 134)
Age (years)	62 ± 11	63 ± 10
Gender: Female	19%	22%
Race: Caucasian	75%	72%
NYHA: Class III	93%	95%
MLWHF QOL Score	53 ± 24	52 ± 24
6 min Hall Walk Distance (m)*	316 ± 68	294 ± 73
HR (bpm)	75 ± 10	75 ± 11
SBP (mm Hg)	120 ± 17	121 ± 16
DBP (mm Hg)	73 ± 10	73 ± 10
LVEF (%)	27 ± 7	28 ± 6
NT-pro BNP (pg/mL, median [IQR])	731 [475, 1021]	765 [479, 1052]
eGFR (mL/min)	64 ± 17	62 ± 20
QRS interval	109 ± 18	110 ± 26
History of atrial fibrillation	29%	43%
History of coronary artery disease	62%	69%
Previous HF hospitalization	42%	51%

No significant difference between BAT and control: none below 0.01, 6MHW *P* = .015, AF *P* = .03, all others greater than 0.05.
Abbreviations: DBP, diastolic blood pressure; eGFR, estimated glomerular filtration rate; HR, heart rate; SBP, systolic blood pressure.

Table 2
Baroreflex activation therapy for heart failure baseline therapies for premarket phase

Variables	BAT (n = 130)	Control (n = 134)
Number of meds	3.9 ± 1.2	4.1 ± 1.4
ACE-I/ARB/ARNI	89%	84%
Beta-blocker	95%	95%
MRA	49%	42%
Diuretic	85%	87%
Ivabradine	2%	5%
ICD	78%	79%

No significant difference between BAT and control.

of patients who improved at 6 months compared with baseline was 52% for 1 class improvement and 13% for 2 class improvement, $P < .001$. These results are supported by objective evidence of significant reduction of NT-proBNP. At 6 months after

randomization, NT-proBNP decreased in BAT versus control by 25%. A clinically meaningful improvement is considered 10% or greater.

The results presented above were consistent across a number of important patient subgroups, including atrial fibrillation, sex, and ejection fraction (**Fig. 6**). The BeAT-HF intended for use in population was 20% female and despite documentation of poorer baseline QoL compared with male, the females had similar improvements with BAT in 6MHW, QoL, and NYHA class.[18] In fact, female individuals had a more significant improvement in NT-proBNP levels compared with male, suggesting that female are likely to benefit from BAT at least as much as male, if not more.

In the Pre-Market phase of BeAT-HF, BAT was shown to be safe in patients with HFrEF as measured by the Major Adverse Neurological or Cardiovascular system or procedure-related event rate (MANCE). The MANCE free rate was 97%, $P < .001$.

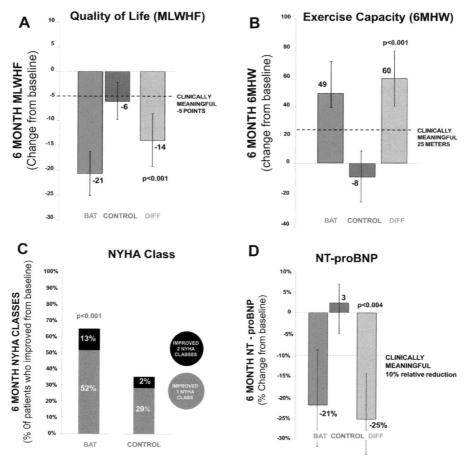

Fig. 5. Effects of 6 months of BAT on patient-centered symptom status. (*A*) *QoL*: assessed using the MLWHFQ. (*B*) *Exercise capacity*: assessed using the 6MHWD. *Functional status*: assessed by (*C*) the NYHA functional class and (*D*) NT-proBNP. ([*A, B*] *From* Zile MR, Lindenfeld J, Weaver FA, et al. Baroreflex Activation Therapy in Patients With Heart Failure With Reduced Ejection Fraction. J Am Coll Cardiol. 2020;76(1):1-13.)

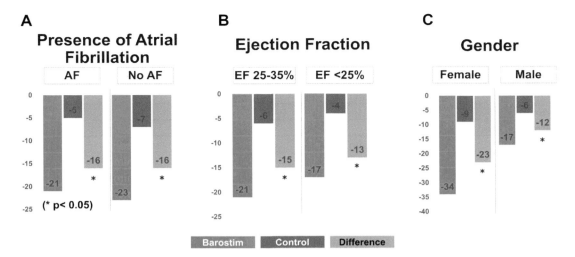

Consistency across subgroups: Health Status (MLWHF)

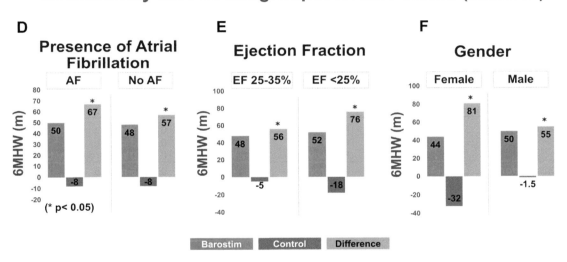

Consistency across subgroups: 6MHW

Fig. 6. Consistency of premarket phase of BeAT-HF results at 6 months across patient subgroups. (*A–C*) Effects of 6 months of BAT on quality of life using the MLWHFQ on patient subgroups with/without atrial fibrillation, ejection fraction 25.025%, less than 25%, male/female sex. (*D–F*) *Effects of 6 months of BAT on exercise capacity*: assessed using the 6 MHWD on patient subgroups with/without atrial fibrillation, ejection fraction 25.025%, less than 25%, male/female sex. (*From* Lindenfeld J, Gupta R, Grazette L, et al. Response by Sex in Patient-Centered Outcomes With Baroreflex Activation Therapy in Systolic Heart Failure. JACC Heart Fail. 2021;9(6):430-438.)

On the basis of all of the data discussed above, the FDA approved BAT on August 16, 2019, with the following instruction for use: The BAROSTIM NEO System is indicated for the improvement of symptoms of HF—QoL, 6MHW, and functional status, for patients who remain symptomatic despite treatment with guideline-directed medical therapy, are NYHA Class III or Class II (who had a recent history of Class III), have a LVEF ≤ 35%, an NT-proBNP less than 1600 pg/mL and excluding patients indicated for CRT according to AHA/ACC/ESC guidelines.

Baroreflex Activation Therapy Surgical Insertion and Titration

The BAT device should be implanted by a surgeon who has familiarity with carotid anatomy and

Table 3
Effects of anesthetic agents on the baroreflex activation therapy and half life of effect

Anesthetic agent	Half life	Effect on the baroreflex
Fentanyl	IV 10–20 min	Preserve
Remifentanil	1–20 min	Preserve
Etomidate	75 min	Preserve
Nitrous Oxide	5 min	Preserve
Rocuronium	66–80 min	Preserve
Midazolam	1.5–2.5 h	Minimally blunt
Thiopental	1.5–2.5 h	Minimally blunt
Isoflurane	10.0 ± 5.57 min	Blunt
Desflurane	8.16 ± 3.15 min	Blunt
Sevoflurane	9.47 ± 4.46 min	Blunt
Propofol	2–3 min; Elimination ½ life 30–60 min	Blunt
Dexmedetomidine	6 min	Blunt
Ketamine	2.5–3 h	Blunt

Table 4
Total Intravenous Anesthesia using Fentanyl

Step of implantation	Anesthetic agent	Suggested dosage
Induction	Midazolam	0.1–0.2 mg/kg
	Etomidate	0.2–0.3 mg/kg
	Fentanyl	0.5–2.0 mcg/kg via IV bolus*
Intubation	Rocuronium	0.3–0.6 mg/kg
Phase I: Lead placement	Midazolam	0.1–0.4 mg/kg/h
	Fentanyl	1.0–2.0 mcg/kg/h
	Morphine	As needed
Phase II: IPG placement	Convert to standard	

Table 5
Total Intravenous Anesthesia using Remifentanil

Step of Implantation	Anesthetic agent	Suggested dosage
Induction	Midazolam	0.1–0.2 mg/kg
	Etomidate	0.2–0.3 mg/kg
	Remifentanil	0.5–1.0 mcg/kg via IV bolus*
Intubation	Rocuronium	0.3–0.6 mg/kg
Phase I: Lead Placement	Midazolam	0.1–0.4 mg/kg/h
	Remifentanil	0.1–0.5 mcg/kg/min
Phase II: IPG Placement	Convert to standard	

Consider administration with infusion pump or syringe driver rather than bolus.
Physicians should use their judgment and knowledge of the patient to determine dosages.

nearby neck structures (internal jugular vein, vagal nerve, hypoglossal nerve, etc) to minimize complications and optimize patient benefit. Surgical evaluation should begin with an assessment of the patient's symptoms and prospective opportunities for improvement of these symptoms with BAT. Neck mobility should be confirmed, particularly in the lateral and posterior directions. Pre-operative carotid duplex ultrasound must be completed and confirm less than 50% stenosis in the internal carotid artery (ICA) ipsilateral to the planned implantation.

Because the intra-operative protocol includes mapping to confirm the location of the carotid body, medications must be modified to prevent inhibition of the baroreflex. First, anti-hypertensives (β-blockers, ACEi, ARB, ARNI, calcium channel blockers, etc) should be held for 24 to 48 hours prior to the procedure. Novel oral anti-coagulants (Eliquis, Xarelto) should be held for 72 hours. Coumadin should be held for 5 days to ensure safe and hemostatic surgical field. Aspirin may be continued throughout the peri-operative period and surgeon choice impacts the decision regarding temporary cessation of additional anti-platelet agents (Plavix, Brilinta, etc). With the

addition of SGLT2 inhibitors to guideline-directed medical therapies for HF, it is important that the peri-operative team identifies and holds these medications for 48 hours prior to surgery to avoid euglycemic ketoacidosis post-operatively. To minimize the risk of volume overload, it is advisable to continue diuretics throughout the peri-operative period. Medications can typically be resumed as originally prescribed immediately after the procedure.

A list of preferred anesthetic agents has been compiled to minimize patient recall while allowing for accurate and sensitive assessment of the baroreflex (**Table 3**). Two common protocols have also been included for clarification (**Tables 4** and **5**). After placement of arterial line and induction of anesthesia, the patient is positioned with a shoulder-roll to lengthen the neck and with the head turned away from the implantation site (typically right side when able). Transverse neck incision over the carotid bifurcation (as mapped in the OR by ultrasound by the operative surgeon) allows for adequate exposure while minimizing injury to cranial nerves (**Fig. 7**). Surgical experience gained during the BEAT-HF trial confirmed safety and informed optimal exposure (see

BAT Implant Technique

Small Incision in Neck	Electrode sutured to Carotid Artery	Lead tunneled to pectoral pocket	
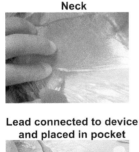	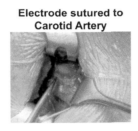	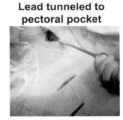	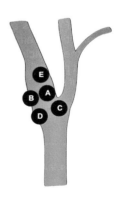
Lead connected to device and placed in pocket	Incision in neck closed	Pocket incision closed	
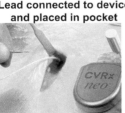	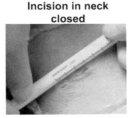	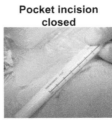	

Requires no leads in the heart or vasculature

Fig. 7. Surgical steps required for BAT implantation and anatomical locations for placement. An incision centered on the carotid bifurcation is made just large enough to expose the anterior surface. The mapping tool is manually guided to establish the optimal electrode location. Once determined, the electrode is fixed with sutures placed around the perimeter of the electrode backer. Mapping occurred in recommended sequence A–E on the internal carotid artery and carotid bifurcation. If no anterior location was determined to be suitable, mapping may be continued on the posterior surface. (*From* Weaver FA, Abraham WT, Little WC, et al. Surgical Experience and Long-term Results of Baroreflex Activation Therapy for Heart Failure With Reduced Ejection Fraction. Semin Thorac Cardiovasc Surg. 2016;28(2):320-328.)

Components of Baroreflex Activation Therapy (BAT) Device

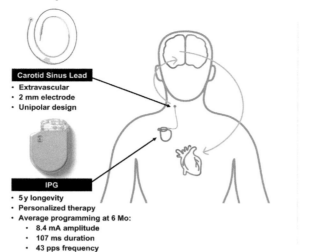

Carotid Sinus Lead
- Extravascular
- 2 mm electrode
- Unipolar design

IPG
- 5 y longevity
- Personalized therapy
- Average programming at 6 Mo:
  - 8.4 mA amplitude
  - 107 ms duration
  - 43 pps frequency

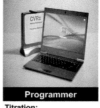

Programmer

Titration:
- 8.4 mA amplitude
- 107 ms duration
- 43 pps frequency

Fig. 8. Components of the BAT device. IPG, implantable pulse generator.

Fig. 7) as well as positioning on the vessels such that the inner curvature of the carotid bifurcation (sites A + C) was responsive in nearly 80% of patients (see **Fig. 7**; **Fig. 8**).[19] Position confirmation is tested by activating the device and detecting greater than 10% decrease in heart rate and/or greater than 5% decrease in BP. The device is maintained in place and the stimulation is stopped to confirm a "rebound" effect to baseline. Each of these steps should occur within 60 seconds to have confidence that the carotid body has been targeted. The device is tacked with peri-adventitial sutures and the lead is then tunneled through the sternocleidomastoid muscle and across the clavicle to join the battery secured in the chest pocket. Incisional care is surgeon preference, but utilization of subcuticular closure and coverage with skin glue is common. Postoperative surveillance for bleeding, stroke, and

BP issues may occur in the recovery area for 2 to 4 hours prior to the patient's safe discharge to home. The patient typically should leave the hospital with the device turned on at 1 mA. The first titration will often occur at about 2 weeks such that the device amplitude is increased until the patient feels any electrical stimulation in the neck muscle or skin, then the stimulation is reduced for comfort. Titrations may occur every 2 to 4 weeks based on patient response to the therapy with a goal of reaching optimized therapy by 6 months (**Table 6**).

FUTURE DIRECTIONS

In the post-market phase of BeAT-HF, the primary endpoint will be a composite of cardiovascular (CV) mortality and HF morbidity and the additional pre-specified endpoints listed in **Fig. 9**. This will be an intention to treat analysis, that will include 323

Table 6
Baroreflex activation therapy titration

Visit	Amplitude (mA)		Frequency (pps)		Pulse Width (ms)	
	N	Mean ± SD	N	Mean ± SD	N	Mean ± SD
Implant	120	1.4 ± 0.5	120	48.5 ± 16.3	120	143.9 ± 23.7
Month 0.5	105	3.5 ± 1.0	105	48.4 ± 15.6	105	145.5 ± 25.1
Month 1	103	5.0 ± 1.5	103	47.0 ± 14.2	103	135.2 ± 33.8
Month 1.5	98	6.3 ± 1.8	98	47.0 ± 14.0	98	130.1 ± 35.8
Month 2	102	7.1 ± 2.0	102	46.7 ± 13.7	102	122.4 ± 37.4
Month 3	100	7.7 ± 2.3	100	46.0 ± 13.8	100	114.5 ± 38.6
Month 6	120	8.3 ± 2.4	120	43.6 ± 12.2	120	109.1 ± 37.5

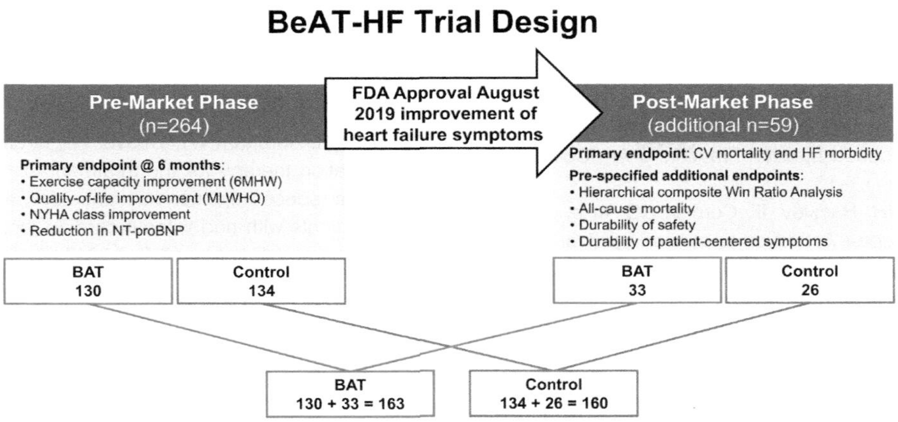

BeAT-HF Trial Design

Fig. 9. BeAT-HF trial design.

randomized patients. These data are expected to be published in 2023.

In addition, development of percutaneous delivery system for the BAT lead has been developed and is being tested in the BATwire Trial (NCT04600791).

CLINICS CARE POINTS

- In patients with NYHA Class III HFrEF who have already received maximally tolerated GDMT, patient-centered symptomatic improvement can be achieved with BAT.

- BAT can be personalized for each patient with HFrEF because the strength of stimulation can be modified at any time for any circumstance.

- All device components of BAT are extravascular; thus avoiding potential complications of other intravascular devices used in the treatment of HFrEF.

DISCLOSURES

All authors have disclosures as follows:

Drs J.M. Ruddy, A. Kroman, and M.R. Zile served as consultants to CVRx. Dr C.F. Baicu has nothing to disclose.

ACKNOWLEDGMENTS

None.

REFERENCES

1. Floras JS. Sympathetic nervous system activation in human heart failure: clinical implications of an updated model. J Am Coll Cardiol 2009;54(5): 375–85.
2. Creager MA, Creager SJ. Arterial baroreflex regulation of blood pressure in patients with congestive heart failure. J Am Coll Cardiol 1994;23(2):401–5.
3. Mortara A, La Rovere MT, Pinna GD, et al. Arterial baroreflex modulation of heart rate in chronic heart failure: clinical and hemodynamic correlates and prognostic implications. Circulation 1997;96(10): 3450–8.
4. Giannoni A, Gentile F, Buoncristiani F, et al. Chemoreflex and Baroreflex Sensitivity Hold a Strong Prognostic Value in Chronic Heart Failure. JACC Heart Fail 2022;10(9):662–76.
5. Yancy CW, Jessup M, Bozkurt B, et al. 2013 ACCF/AHA guideline for the management of heart failure: a report of the American College of Cardiology Foundation/American Heart Association Task Force on Practice Guidelines. Circulation 2013;128:e240–327.
6. Yancy CW, Jessup M, Bozkurt B, et al. 2017 ACC/AHA/HFSA focused update of the 2013 ACCF/AHA guideline for the management of heart failure: a report of the American College of Cardiology/American Heart Association Task Force on Clinical Practice Guidelines and the Heart Failure Society of America. Circulation 2017;136:e137–61.
7. Heidenreich PA, Bozkurt B, Aguilar D, et al. 2022 AHA/ACC/HFSA Guideline for the Management of Heart Failure: A Report of the American College of Cardiology/American Heart Association Joint Committee on Clinical Practice Guidelines. Circulation 2022;145(18):e895–1032.
8. Gronda E, Seravalle G, Brambilla G, et al. Chronic baroreflex activation effects on sympathetic nerve traffic, baroreflex function, and cardiac haemodynamics in heart failure: a proof-of-concept study. Eur J Heart Fail 2014;16(9):977–83.
9. Wustmann K, Kucera JP, Scheffers I, et al. Effects of chronic baroreceptor stimulation on the autonomic

cardiovascular regulation in patients with drug-resistant arterial hypertension. Hypertension 2009; 54(3):530–6.

10. Zile MR, Lindenfeld J, Weaver FA, et al. Baroreflex Activation Therapy in Patients With Heart Failure With Reduced Ejection Fraction. J Am Coll Cardiol 2020;76(1):1–13.

11. Zucker IH, Hackley JF, Cornish KG, et al. Chronic Baroreceptor Activation Enhances Survival in Dogs With Pacing-Induced Heart Failure. Hypertension 2007;50(5):904–10.

12. Sabbah HN, Gupta RC, Imai M, et al. Chronic Electrical Stimulation of the Carotid Sinus Baroreflex Improves Left Ventricular Function and Promotes Reversal of Ventricular Remodeling in Dogs With Advanced Heart Failure. Circ Heart Fail 2011;4(1): 65–70.

13. de Leeuw PW, Alnima T, Lovett E, et al. Bilateral or Unilateral Stimulation for Baroreflex Activation Therapy. Hypertension 2015;65(1):187–92.

14. Bisognano JD, Bakris G, Nadim MK, et al. Baroreflex Activation Therapy Lowers Blood Pressure in Patients With Resistant Hypertension. J Am Coll Cardiol 2011;58(7):765–73.

15. Abraham WT, Zile MR, Weaver FA, et al. Baroreflex Activation Therapy for the Treatment of Heart Failure With a Reduced Ejection Fraction. JACC Heart Fail 2015;3(6):487–96.

16. Zile MR, Abraham WT, Weaver FA, et al. Baroreflex activation therapy for the treatment of heart failure with a reduced ejection fraction: safety and efficacy in patients with and without cardiac resynchronization therapy. Eur J Heart Fail 2015;17(10):1066–74.

17. Zile MR, Abraham WT, Lindenfeld J, et al. First granted example of novel FDA trial design under Expedited Access Pathway for premarket approval: BeAT-HF. Am Heart J 2018;204:139–50.

18. Lindenfeld J, Gupta R, Grazette L, et al. Response by Sex in Patient-Centered Outcomes With Baroreflex Activation Therapy in Systolic Heart Failure. JACC Heart Fail 2021;9(6):430–8.

19. Weaver FA, Abraham WT, Little WC, et al. Surgical Experience and Long-term Results of Baroreflex Activation Therapy for Heart Failure With Reduced Ejection Fraction. Semin Thorac Cardiovasc Surg 2016;28(2):320–8.

Cardiac Contractility Modulation
Implications in Heart Failure, a Current Review

Alexander L. Wallner, MD, Salvatore Savona, MD, Rami Kahwash, MD*

KEYWORDS

• Cardiac contractility modulation • Heart failure • Implantable device • Optimizer • Cardiomyopathy

KEY POINTS

- Cardiac contractility modulation (CCM) is Food and Drug Administration (FDA) approved for treatment of heart failure patients with left ventricular ejection fraction (LVEF) between 25% and 45% with persistent symptoms on optimal medical therapy who are not a candidate for CRT.
- Further research investigates expanded inclusion criteria for CCM with a wider range of LVEF including patient with midrange and preserved ejection fraction.
- Future device may include CCM combination capability with implantable cardiac defibrillator.

INTRODUCTION

Heart disease is the leading cause of death in the United States.[1] Heart failure is estimated to affect 6.2 million patients in the United States and causes up to 400,000 deaths annually.[2] This is a common cause of hospital admissions, with significant associated morbidity and mortality,[3] with an estimated cost of US$30.7 billion to the US economy. Heart failure management has made many improvements in the past several decades and at this time consists of pharmacologic and device-based therapy. Pharmacologic therapy is now referred to as the "4 pillars" of heart failure therapy, with angiotensin-converting enzyme inhibitors/angiotensin receptor blockers, beta blockers, mineralocorticoid receptor antagonists (MRA), and sodium-glucose cotransported-2 inhibitors (SGLT2i). The past decade has seen several advancements in medical therapy including the approval of angiotensin-neprilysin inhibitors (Entresto),[4] ivabradine,[5] and SGLT2i[6] for the management of chronic heart failure.

Along with optimal medical therapy, there are important device therapies that have been shown to improve quality of life and overall mortality. Implantable cardioverter-defibrillators are approved in select heart failure patients with reduced LVEF and have been down to decrease overall and cardiovascular death in this group.[7,8] Among heart failure patients with cardiac conduction system disease, cardiac resynchronization therapy (CRT) has been shown to reduce mortality and improve functional capacity while reducing hospitalizations in select populations. Although many patients can benefit from CRT therapy, it is estimated that only 1 in 3 heart failure patients qualify for this therapy.[9] Recently, novel device therapeutics for heart failure have emerged in the form of cardiac contractility modulation (CCM).

CCM, delivered by the Optimizer Smart and Optimizer Smart Mini devices produced by Impulse Dynamics (Marlton, NJ, USA), uses nonexcitatory cardiac stimulations to enhance cardiac contractility. This increase in contractility provides a benefit to cardiac output and improves hemodynamics in heart failure patients on top of optimal pharmacotherapy to ultimately lead to improved patient outcomes. In this review, we will discuss implementation of CCM from device implantation,

Division of Cardiovascular Medicine, The Ohio State University Wexner Medical Center, Columbus, OH, USA
* Corresponding author. Davis Heart & Lung Research Institute, 473 West 12th Avenue, Suite 200, Columbus, OH 43210.
E-mail address: rami.kahwash@osumc.edu

Heart Failure Clin 20 (2024) 51–60
https://doi.org/10.1016/j.hfc.2023.05.006
1551-7136/24/© 2023 Elsevier Inc. All rights reserved.

heartfailure.theclinics.com

physiologic mechanism, current evidence, and patient qualifications along with future developments for possible expansion of use in various patient populations.

DEVICE OVERVIEW
Device Function

The CCM device is a cardiac implanted device, consisting of a pulse generator connected to 2 (or 3) intracardiac leads.[10] Typically, the generator is implanted in the subcutaneous tissue below the clavicle with leads entering through the subclavian vein with tips implanted in the right ventricular septum. The battery is charged via a transcutaneous system (**Fig. 1**), as opposed to serial invasive battery changes in standard implanted pacemaker/defibrillator systems. CCM therapy uses biphasic electrical stimulation at relatively high voltages (7.5 V) applied to the ventricular endocardium during the absolute refractory period of the cardiac action potential (**Fig. 2**).[11] By stimulating in the absolute refractory period, this impulse does not generate a new action potential. CCM therapy is typically activated for up to 12 hours daily and can be adjusted as needed based on patient and physician preference.[11] In the United States, CCM therapy is approved to be delivered during 5 1-hour therapy delivery phases separated by 3.8-hour therapy-off periods. In the latest generation devices (ie, Smart Mini), duration of therapy intervals can be increased to ensure greater than 90% treated QRS complexes to account for the device withholding therapy during ectopic beats and tachyarrhythmias. Earlier clinical work showed that delivery of CCM therapy is equally safe and seems similarly effective over the range of shorter (5 hours) to longer (12 hours) periods daily according to one study.[12] Optimizer

Smart and mini are MRI compatible and safe to be used with personal electronic devices. Of note, some newer personal electronic devices such as iPhones have a magnet in their device body, and therefore, if placed close to the Smart Mini will place the device in Magnet Mode—which suspends therapies for 24 hours.

Device Implantation

Implantation of a CCM device is similar to implantation of a transvenous leaded device such as a pacemaker or a defibrillator. A preprocedure evaluation should consider if the patient has a preexisting transvenous device, the potential for needing another transvenous device such as a defibrillator, the handedness of the patient, and if the patient has any earlier surgeries or radiation therapy near the procedure site. Given the fact that many patients have left ventricular systolic dysfunction and may require a transvenous defibrillator in the future, a right-sided implant is typically performed. Leads from any manufacturer can be used for device implant, per operator preference. The leads are implanted into the intraventricular septum at least 2 cm apart. As both leads are implanted into the intraventricular septum, preformed sheaths that are utilized for conduction system pacing may provide efficient access to the septum. Both leads are tested after implantation in the same manner as if they were implanted for pacing, including assessment of the current of injury, sensing amplitude, pacing impedance, and pacing threshold. If acceptable parameters are met, the CCM device may be attached to the leads in order to test the therapy and ensure the patient does not have discomfort from the therapy, which has been reported as a "rattling" or "vibrating" sensation in the chest. If a preformed sheath is

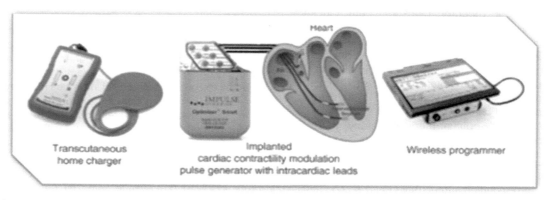

Fig. 1. A transcutaneous home charger, an implanted device, and a wireless programmer used during implant are shown. (*From* Campbell CM, Kahwash R, Abraham WT. Optimizer Smart in the treatment of moderate-to-severe chronic heart failure. Future Cardiol. 2020;16(1):13-25.)

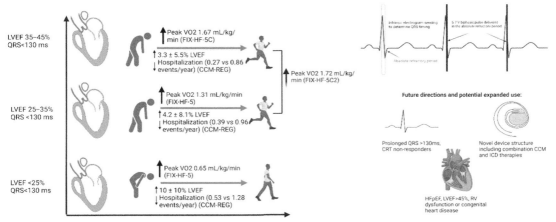

Fig. 2. Cardiac contractility modulation: implementation and efficacy in heart failure patients. (*Created with* BioRender.com.)

used, this testing may be performed before slitting the sheaths in the event the leads need to be repositioned to avoid this sensation. If the leads are in an acceptable location, they may be secured in a similar fashion to a standard pacing lead. The device may be reattached to the leads, and the pocket closed. Following the procedure, a chest X-ray should be performed to ensure there are no complications with lead insertion, such as a pneumothorax, and to assess stable lead position. **Fig. 3** below shows an example of a postprocedure chest X-ray in a patient who had a prior single

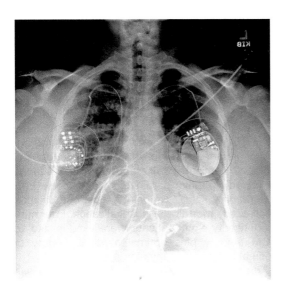

Fig. 3. Postoperative chest radiograph of a left-sided single chamber ICD (*red circle*), right-sided CCM device (*blue circle*), and leads for CCM therapy (*yellow arrows*). (*From* Tang JE, Ryu JN, Essandoh MK, Savona SJ. Two Implantable Devices for Cardiac Rhythm Management. J Cardiothorac Vasc Anesth. 2023;37(2):326-329.)

chamber left-sided transvenous defibrillator, and a right-sided CCM device.

MECHANISM OF ACTION

CCM uses nonexcitatory stimulation of cardiac myocytes during the absolute refractory period of cardiac muscle. The mechanism of action is multilayered and likely mediated by enhanced myocardial intercellular calcium handling, which leads to an increase in contractility. This acute and temporarily increased contractility has been demonstrated in vitro and in vivo animal and human studies. Further studies have demonstrated improved cardiac gene expression and structural reverse remodeling after CCM therapy.[13]

- *Improved contractility and LV function:* In isolated rabbit right ventricular (RV) papillary muscle nonexcitatory electrical stimulation was found to modulate the action potential duration and enhance contractility.[14] These findings were reproduced in in vitro samples of failing human trabeculae muscle. In a dog model of heart failure, LVEF increased from 31% to 41% ($P<.05$) after only 6 hours of CCM therapy.[15] In humans, 3 months of CCM therapy was shown to increase LVEF (4.8 $\pm$ 3.6%, $P<.001$) through an increase in global and regional contractility.[16] CCM has also been shown to decrease global longitudinal strain and increased LV mechanical performance through echocardiographic measurement of mechano-energetic efficiency (32.2 $\pm$ 10.1 vs 38.6 $\pm$ 7.6 mL/s; $P = .013$).[17] Importantly, the increase in LV contractility seen with CCM is not associated with an increase in myocardial oxygen demand.[18]

- *Enhanced calcium handling:* The improvement in cardiac contractility by CCM seems to be calcium dependent as shown by the following studies. In 2001, CCM was shown to increase intracellular calcium in isolated, superfused, isometrically contracting rabbit papillary muscles by aequorin luminescence technique.[19] The increase in contractility was attenuated by ryanodine[19] and verapamil,[14] further supporting the calcium-dependent mechanism.

- *Structural reverse remodeling:* Along with enhanced calcium handling, CCM has been shown to effect myocardial cell structure. The protein titin acts as a spring in structural support to the cardiomyocyte.[20] Titin expression is altered by phosphorylation. In a dog model of heart failure, cytoskeletal titin is reduced, and this level is returned to normal after CCM therapy.[21] In a rabbit model of congestive heart failure (CHF), CCM has been shown to reduce structural and electrical remodeling as shown by a decreased hydroxyproline content and attenuated a decrease in Kv4.3, KCNQ1, KCNH2, and Cx43 protein levels (markers of electrical dysfunction).[22]

- *Gene expression:* Alteration in cellular gene expression is seen in heart failure. CCM therapy has been shown to attenuate these maladaptive gene expression changes.[23] In one study, the upregulation of the myocardial fetal gene program and stretch response genes along with downregulation of calcium handling genes was reversed after 3 months of CCM therapy.[24]

EVIDENCE FOR UTILIZATION OF CARDIAC CONTRACTILITY MODULATION
Initial Studies

Pilot study

The first major randomized clinical trial involving CCM was published in 2006 by Neelagaru and colleagues (**Table 1**). This study enrolled heart failure patients with reduced LVEF of 35% or lesser with the New York Heart Association (NYHA) class III or IV symptoms. Patients had to be treated with stable doses of optimal medical therapy, as well as have an implantable cardiac defibrillator (ICD) in place. The presence of CRT device, atrial fibrillation, or a high burden of premature ventricular contractions (PVCs) (>8900/24 h as measured by Holter monitor) were exclusion criteria. Forty-nine patients were enrolled in the trial, and all patients had the 3-lead CCM system implanted. After randomization, 25 patients had CCM therapy

turned on, whereas the others were left off. In the CCM therapy arm, the primary safety endpoint was achieved with less hospitalizations (62% vs 84%) in comparison to the control arm. CCM therapy trended toward improved clinical outcomes with increases in peak Vo_2, 6-min walk and anaerobic threshold, although the improvement did not reach statistical significance.[25]

FIX-HF4

In 2008, the FIX-HF-4 trial was published, which further investigated the efficacy of CCM therapy. This was a randomized, double-blind, cross-over study with primary endpoints of improved functional capacity as measured by peak Vo_2 score, and quality of life, as measured by Minnesota Living with Heart Failure Questionnaire (MLHFQ) scores. Patients with symptomatic heart failure with LVEF35% or lesser and peak Vo_2 between 10 and 20 mL/kg/min were included. Patients were not required to have an ICD implanted. The presence of a CRT device, atrial fibrillation, or a high burden of PVCs (>8900/24 h as measured by Holter monitor) were exclusion criteria. The trial was positive in favor of CCM therapy with a significant increase in peak Vo_2 (0.99 mL/kg/min, $P = .03$) and a decrease in the Minnesota living with heart failure questionnaire (MLWHFQ) scores. There was no increase in adverse events such as PVCs or ICD discharge seen with CCM therapy.[26]

FIX-HF5

The clinical efficacy of CCM therapy was further demonstrated in the HF-5C trial in 2011 by Kadish and colleagues.[27] This trial aimed to demonstrate a benefit in clinical heart failure outcomes along with device safety. The primary endpoint was an improvement in exercise capacity as measured by ventilatory anaerobic threshold (VAT) increase of more than 20%. Patients with an LVEF of 35% or lesser and poor functional capacity as defined by NYHA class III or IV and peak Vo_2 of 9 mL/kg/min or greater were enrolled. Secondary endpoints included 6-minute walk test, MHLHFQ scores, echocardiographic parameters, and peak Vo_2. The primary safety endpoint was a combination of all-cause mortality or hospitalization. Four hundred twenty-eight patients were randomized to CCM therapy plus optimal medical therapy or optimal medical therapy along.

The primary safety endpoint was met, along with a significant increase in peak Vo_2 values in the CCM therapy group (0.65 mL/kg/min, $P = .024$). The primary endpoint of a significant increase in VAT was not met. Patients did report an increase in quality of life, with a change in MLHFQ score of -9.7 ($P<.0001$). The increase in exercise

Table 1
Summary of cardiac contractility modulation trials

	Number of Participants	Study Design	Inclusion Criteria	Primary Endpoint	Secondary Endpoints
Pilot study (2006)	49	Prospective, randomized trial	LVEF ≤35%, NYHA class III/IV symptoms on optimal GDMT. QRS <130 ms	• Reduction in hospitalizations (62% vs 84%)	• Trend toward increase in peak VO_2, 6-min walk, anaerobic threshold
FIX-HF-4 (2008)	164	Prospective, randomized, double-blind cross-over trial	LVEF ≤35%, peak VO_2 10–20 mL/kg/min, on optimal GDMT. QRS <130 ms	• Increase in peak VO_2 of 0.99 mL/kg/min ($P = .03$)	• No increase in arrhythmia, PVC, or ICD shock with device therapy
FIX-HF-5 (2011)	428	Prospective, randomized trial	LVEF ≤35%, NYHA class III/IV symptoms, peak VO_2 >9 mL/kg/min on optimal GDMT. QRS <130 ms	• No significant increase in VAT • No increase in adverse events (hospitalization or mortality)	• Increase in peak VO_2 of 0.65 mL/kg/min ($P = .024$) • Increase in quality of life (MNLHFQ score of −9.7 $P<.0001$)
FIX-HF-5C (2018)	160	Prospective, randomized, unblinded trial	LVEF ≥25% and ≤45%, persistent symptoms on optimal GDMT. QRS<130 ms	• Increase in peak VO_2 of 0.84 mL/kg/min (95% Bayesian credible interval: 0.123–1.552)	• Increase in MNLHFQ score, NYHA class, and 6-min walk
FIX-HF-5C2(2020)	60	Prospective nonrandomized single arm, comparison to control arm of FIX-HF-5C trial	LVEF ≥25% and ≤45%, persistent symptoms on optimal GDMT. QRS <130 ms	• Similar CCM delivery efficacy between 2 and 3 lead systems • Similar safety profile between 2 and 3 lead systems	• Improvement in NYHA functional class (83% vs 43%, $P < .0001$) • Improvement in peak VO_2 at 12 and 24 wk
CCM-Registry(2021)	503	Prospective observational study of CCM registry	LVEF ≤45%, included patients with LVEF ≤25% and those with atrial fibrillation	• Improvement in NYHA functional class (0.6 ± 0.7, $P<.001$)	• Decrease in heart failure hospitalization (0.25 from 0.74 admissions/y, $P<.0001$). • Estimated overall 1 y and 3 y survival by MAGIC risk score

capacity was more notable in patients with a moderate range of systolic dysfunction with an increase of peak Vo_2 of 1.31 mL/kg/min (P<.0001) in patients with LVEF 25% to 35%, suggesting that patients were severe LV dysfunction may not benefit as much from the device.[27]

FIX-HF5C

In response to the FIX-HF5 study, the FIX-HF-5C study was designed, which aimed to confirm the earlier findings that suggested clinical improvement with CCM in patients with LVEF between 25% and 45%. FIX-HF-5C was a prospective randomized study of 160 patients investigating the effect of CCM compared with optimal medical therapy in patients with LVEF of 25% or greater and 45% or lesser with QRS less than 130 milliseconds. There was a significant improvement in the primary endpoint of exercise tolerance with peak Vo_2 increase of 0.84 mL/kg/min (95% Bayesian credible interval: 0.123–1.552). Quality of life metrics also were significantly improved as measured by MLHFQ score, NYHA class, and 6-minute walk. There were 7 device-related complications, reaching the primary safety endpoint of 80% of patients remaining complication free. A 7.9% absolute reduction in cardiovascular mortality and heart failure hospitalization was found (P = .048).[28]

Follow-up Trials

CCM-REG

The above trials, including FIX-HF5C, demonstrated clinical improvement with CCM therapy during 6 months follow-up. Subsequently, the CCM-Registry was developed to follow patients with CCM chronically. Data for the initial 140 patients in the registry was published in 2019, with 3 years of follow-up. Patients were divided into 2 cohorts with LVEF 25% to 34% (CCM-Reg25-34, 83 patients) and LVEF 35% to 45% (CCM-REG35-45, 57 patients). CCM-REG25-34 demonstrated a significant 75% reduction in hospitalization (1.2/patient-year compared with 0.35/patient-year, P <.0001) with improvement in MLHFQ scores and 6-minute walk times. Overall mortality as compared with the Seattle Heart Failure Model was comparable. CCM-REG35-45 demonstrated similar improvement in hospitalization, MLHFQ, and 6-minute walk times. However, a significant improvement in 3-year survival was noted (88.0% vs 74.7%, P = .046).[29]

In 2021, a repeat analysis of the CCM registry was released. This analysis included 503 patients from 51 European countries. In comparison to the earlier study performed in 2019, this study included patients with LVEF less than 25% and those with atrial fibrillation. All subgroups of LVEF demonstrated an improvement in NYHA class (0.6 ± 0.7, P < .001), MLWHFQ score (10 ± 21, P < .001), and LVEF (5.6 ± 8.4%, P < .001). Heart failure hospitalizations decreased (0.74–0.25 per patient/y, P < .0001). Estimated overall survival over 1 and 3 years predicted by MAGGIC risk score was improved in all subgroups as well. Patients with atrial fibrillation demonstrated similar improvement to those without.[30]

FIX-HF5C2

The previous studies above used a 3-lead Optimizer Smart CCM system, with an atrial lead and 2 ventricular leads. Subsequently, a 2-lead Optimizer Smart system was developed, which eliminated the need for an atrial lead. The FIX-HF5C2 trial aimed to evaluate the safety and efficacy of the new 2 lead system. Although the prior 3-lead system relied on the detection of atrial activation to time CCM therapy, the 2-lead system does not rely on atrial activation for timing. This allows for utilization in patients with atrial fibrillation. Moreover, because only 2 leads are used, there is a potential for increased safety given a simpler system with fewer leads and less device-related complications.

This study was a single-arm, prospective trial, which enrolled 60 patients with an LVEF between 25% and 45% and NYHA class III or IV symptoms. All patients were treated with optimal doses of medical therapy. Patients were excluded if they qualified for CRT therapy, and ICDs had to be implanted when indicated. Patients with a recent (within 30 days) heart failure hospitalization or utilization of inotrope therapy were excluded. Although not a randomized trial, patients were evaluated clinically during a 24-week follow-up and were compared with the control arm group of the FIX-HF-5C study.

Patients were followed with repeat cardiopulmonary exercise tests and evaluated for device effectiveness as measured by CCM device activations along with safety endpoints as defined as device-related complications. CCM delivery was similar between the 2 and 3 lead systems, with a goal of 5 hours of CCM therapy per 24-hour period. Importantly, there was no decrease in device delivery in patients with permanent atrial fibrillation. Exercise capacity significantly improved in the device therapy group with an increase in peak Vo_2 at 12 weeks (1.08 [95% CI 0.38–1.78] mL/kg/min) and 24 weeks (1.72 [95% CI 1.02–2.42] mL/kg/min). Overall functional class improved in the device therapy group with 83% reporting an improvement in 1 NYHA class compared with 43% in the control group (P < .0001). Only 1 patient (1.7%) experienced a device-related complication during the follow-up period, compared with a 10.3% complication rate in FIX-HF5C.[31]

Cardiac contractility modulation in patients with atrial fibrillation

The initial CCM system algorithms relied on an atrial lead to sense atrial activation in order to time CCM therapy delivery during the absolute refractory period. Due to potential interference with the algorithm, patients with atrial arrhythmias such as atrial fibrillation or atrial flutter were initially excluded from CCM therapy. Then, in small case series, small groups of patients with atrial fibrillation were treated with an altered algorithm, which relied instead on paced atrial stimulation rather than sensing native atrial rhythm.[32] CCM therapy was successful, resulting in improvement in clinical symptoms, although with slightly lower CCM therapy percentage of around 74% of QRS complexes. Later, the 2-lead Optimizer Smart system was released with a redesigned algorithm, which did not rely on atrial sensing for therapy delivery. The FIX-HF-5C2 study tested the feasibility and efficacy of this system. In subgroup analysis, patients with and without atrial fibrillation had similar CCM efficacies.[31] Similar findings were seen in a 2021 review of the CCM-REG registry with similar improvement in clinical outcomes and reduced heart failure hospitalization with CCM therapy in patients with and without atrial fibrillation.[30] In response to these findings, atrial fibrillation as an exclusion was removed from the FDA indication for CCM in October 2021.

EXPANDED USE AND FUTURE DIRECTIONS OF CARDIAC CONTRACTILITY MODULATION
Cardiac Resynchronization Therapy Nonresponders

CRT is approved for patients with moderate-to-severe heart failure with LVEF of 35% or lesser and persistent symptoms with optimal medical therapy with a wide QRS (>130 milliseconds) in a left bundle branch pattern.[33] Patients who met criteria for CRT were not included in the CCM trials above. However, approximately 1 in 3 patients who receive CRT therapy do not have a clinical response and are referred to as CRT nonresponders.[9] These patients may then benefit from CCM therapy. Several recent small case series have shown an increase in NYHA functional class, peak V_{O_2} and MLHFQ scores after CCM implantation in 17 CRT nonresponders.[34] Further studies are needed to investigate the potential benefit of CCM in CRT nonresponders, or even as combination therapy with CRT given the distinct mechanisms of these therapies.

Heart Failure with Preserved Ejection Fraction

Current FDA approval for CCM therapy includes patients with an LVEF between 25% and 45%. In the recent decade, there has been more focus on patients with clinical heart failure and a preserved LVEF, typically defined as LVEF greater than 40%. Recent studies have demonstrated new pharmacologic treatments for this patient cohort, including SGLT2 inhibitors and MRA in certain patients. Device therapy is limited in this group. A recent pilot study of CCM therapy in 47 patients with heart failure with preserved ejection fraction (HFpEF) demonstrated an improvement in Kansas City Cardiomyopathy Questionnaire scores (18.0 ± 16.6 points, $P < .001$) with a good safety profile.[35] Currently, the AIM-HIGHER study is investigating CCM therapy in patients with LVEF between 40% and 60%.

RV Dysfunction and Congenital Heart Disease

There are limited treatment options for patients with right ventricular dysfunction and most current heart failure therapies are primarily efficacious in left ventricular dysfunction. Congenital heart disease is a varied spectrum of anatomical dysfunction but frequently presents with RV dysfunction; therefore, CCM may be a promising new treatment in this field. In a sheep model of repaired Tetralogy of Fallot with RV dysfunction, CCM was shown to increase RV function as evidenced by a significant increase in right ventricular dP/dt ($P<.05$).[36] In a recent study by Contaldi and colleagues, the effects of CCM on RV performance were assessed at 6 months of therapy by echocardiographic criteria.[37] CCM increases metrics of RV reverse remodeling and performance, including reducing RV size and improving RV systolic function, right ventricular systolic pressure (RVSP), and right ventricle (RV)-pulmonary artery (PA) coupling. Treatment options for RV dysfunction are limited, further studies are needed if CCM may be beneficial for these patients.

Combination Device with Implantable Cardiac Defibrillator or Cardiac Resynchronization Therapy

There is significant overlap between patients who qualify and would benefit from ICD protection from SCD and those that could benefit from CCM therapy. Currently, these patients would require 2 separate implanted devices, each with their own set of intracardiac leads. This poses potential problems related to an increased number of devices and leads, including infection and vascular complication such as stenosis and superior vena cava

(SVC) syndrome. Therefore, a combination device with CCM and ICD therapy may be beneficial and is being investigated. As discussed above, CCM therapy has been reserved for patients who do not qualify for CRT therapy. An early study in CCM feasibility demonstrated improved hemodynamics (17.0 +/- 7.5% increase in pulse pressure, P<.01) with CCM in conjunction with biventricular pacing above biventricular pacing alone.[38] Further studies are needed to examine the effect of CCM in conjunction with CRT therapy because these mechanisms are not mutually exclusive.

Cardiac Contractility Modulation and Tricuspid Regurgitation

Tricuspid regurgitation (TR) is a long-term complication that can be caused by all cardiac implantable devices (CIDs) requiring placement of right ventricular endocardial leads such as pacemakers and ICDs. CCM required placement of additional 2 standard pacing leads attached to the RV side of the interventricular septum. Most patients who received CCM therapies in clinic trials were implanted previously with earlier CIDs devices. The effects of transtricuspid leads of CCM and preexisted CIDs on TR severity was evaluated by Masarone and colleagues. In this study, 30 patients indicated for CCM therapy underwent echocardiographic evaluations 24 hours before and 6 months after the Optimizer Smart implant.[17] At the 6-month follow-up, the grade of TR assessed remained unchanged compared with preimplant baseline. The value of the vena contracta and TR proximal isovelocity surface area radius value remained unchanged. CCM enhancement of cardiac contractility and reverse remodeling was thought to be contributing to the preservation of RV geometry and prevention of TR progression. Additionally, chronic RV pacing is a suggested cause of TR associated with CIDs with high percentage pacing capacity is not a concern in CCM therapy because CCM electrical stimulation is nonexcitatory and does not alter the propagation of cardiac impulses.

SUMMARY

CCM is a novel device therapy that improves quality of life and functional capacity in heart failure patients. The device is available to symptomatic patients with LVEF between 25% and 45%, who are not candidates for CRT. Studies have repeatedly shown improvement in functional capacity as assessed by peak Vo_2 and improvement in quality-of-life scores. Some studies have shown a trend toward fewer heart failure hospitalization and even decreased mortality. Originally, patients

with atrial fibrillation were excluded from CCM trials; however, with newer devices not relying on atrial sensing the device may now be used in patients with atrial fibrillation and recent studies suggest similar outcomes in this group. Expanded use may see benefit in patients with prolonged QRS who have not responded to CRT therapy, patients with RV dysfunction and those with mildly reduced or preserved LVEF. Further studies are needed to assess efficacy in these groups. Many patients who qualify for CCM also require an ICD or CRT therapy, thus necessitating multiple implantable devices. A combination device with CCM and ICD or CRT therapy may have technical and safety improvements over a 2-device system. Heart failure is a leading cause of morbidity and mortality and the number of patients living with heart failure is increasing. Many patients have ongoing symptoms even with optimal medical heart failure therapy. CCM can help improve quality of life and clinical outcomes in these patients who have otherwise met the limit of current heart failure therapy.

CLINICS CARE POINTS

- Heart failure affects many patients worldwide and is a leading cause of morbidity, mortality, and health care spending.

- Heart failure treatments have expanded in the recent decades but device therapy such as ICD and CRT are available only to a small segment of patients.

- CCM is an intracardiac implanted device, which delivers nonexcitatory electrical stimulation to improve cardiac function.

- The mechanism of CCM involves improved intracellular calcium handling, improved cellular structure, and altered gene expression, which leads to an improvement in cardiac contractility without an increase in myocardial oxygen demand.

- Currently, CCM is FDA approved for heart failure patients with an LVEF between 25% and 45% with a QRS duration of less than 130 milliseconds.

- Studies of CCM have shown improvement in functional capacity with increase in peak Vo_2 in patients with LVEF between 25% and 45% on optimal medical therapy.

- Expanded CCM indications may include patients with preserved LV function (LVEF >45%), patients with QRS greater than 130 milliseconds who have not responded to CRT, or those with RV dysfunction.

DISCLOSURE

Dr R. Kahwash is consultant of Medtronic, Cardionomic and Impulse Dynamic.

REFERENCES

1. Murphy SL, National Center for Health Statistics (U.S.). Mortality in the United States, 2020. text. U.S. Department of Health and Human Services, Centers for Disease Control and Prevention, National Center for Health Statistics,; 2021:1 online resource (approximately 8 pages). Available at: https://purl.fdlp.gov/GPO/gpo173376 Connect to resourceCDC https://www.cdc.gov/nchs/data/databriefs/db427.pdf Connect to resource. Accessed June 12, 2023.
2. Virani SS, Alonso A, Aparicio HJ, et al. Heart Disease and Stroke Statistics-2021 Update: A Report From the American Heart Association. Circulation 2021;143(8):e254–743.
3. Shah KS, Xu H, Matsouaka RA, et al. Heart Failure With Preserved, Borderline, and Reduced Ejection Fraction: 5-Year Outcomes. J Am Coll Cardiol 2017;70(20):2476–86.
4. McMurray JJ, Packer M, Desai AS, et al. Angiotensin-neprilysin inhibition versus enalapril in heart failure. N Engl J Med 2014;371(11):993–1004.
5. Swedberg K, Komajda M, Böhm M, et al. Ivabradine and outcomes in chronic heart failure (SHIFT): a randomised placebo-controlled study. Lancet 2010;376(9744):875–85.
6. Packer M, Anker SD, Butler J, et al. Cardiovascular and Renal Outcomes with Empagliflozin in Heart Failure. N Engl J Med 2020;383(15):1413–24.
7. Moss AJ, Zareba W, Hall WJ, et al. Prophylactic implantation of a defibrillator in patients with myocardial infarction and reduced ejection fraction. N Engl J Med 2002;346(12):877–83.
8. Al-Khatib SM, Stevenson WG, Ackerman MJ, et al. 2017 AHA/ACC/HRS Guideline for Management of Patients With Ventricular Arrhythmias and the Prevention of Sudden Cardiac Death: A Report of the American College of Cardiology/American Heart Association Task Force on Clinical Practice Guidelines and the Heart Rhythm Society. J Am Coll Cardiol 2018;72(14):e91–220.
9. Lund LH, Jurga J, Edner M, et al. Prevalence, correlates, and prognostic significance of QRS prolongation in heart failure with reduced and preserved ejection fraction. Eur Heart J 2013;34(7):529–39.
10. Barnes A, Campbell C, Weiss R, et al. Cardiac Contractility Modulation in heart Failure: Mechanisms and Clinical Evidence. Curr Treat Options Cardio Med 2020;22. https://doi.org/10.1007/s11936-020-00852-8.
11. Stix G, Borggrefe M, Wolpert C, et al. Chronic electrical stimulation during the absolute refractory period of the myocardium improves severe heart failure. Eur Heart J 2004;25(8):650–5.
12. Kloppe A, Mijic D, Schiedat F, et al. A randomized comparison of 5 versus 12 hours per day of cardiac contractility modulation treatment for heart failure patients: A preliminary report. Cardiol J 2016;23(1):114–9.
13. Kahwash R, Burkhoff D, Abraham WT. Cardiac contractility modulation in patients with advanced heart failure. Expert Rev Cardiovasc Ther 2013;11(5):635–45.
14. Brunckhorst CB, Shemer I, Mika Y, et al. Cardiac contractility modulation by non-excitatory currents: studies in isolated cardiac muscle. Eur J Heart Fail 2006;8(1):7–15.
15. Morita H, Suzuki G, Haddad W, et al. Cardiac contractility modulation with nonexcitatory electric signals improves left ventricular function in dogs with chronic heart failure. J Card Fail 2003;9(1):69–75.
16. Yu CM, Chan JY, Zhang Q, et al. Impact of cardiac contractility modulation on left ventricular global and regional function and remodeling. JACC Cardiovasc Imaging 2009;2(12):1341–9.
17. Masarone D, Kittleson MM, De Vivo S, et al. The Effects of Device-Based Cardiac Contractility Modulation Therapy on Left Ventricle Global Longitudinal Strain and Myocardial Mechano-Energetic Efficiency in Patients with Heart Failure with Reduced Ejection Fraction. J Clin Med 2022;(19):11.
18. Butter C, Wellnhofer E, Schlegl M, et al. Enhanced inotropic state of the failing left ventricle by cardiac contractility modulation electrical signals is not associated with increased myocardial oxygen consumption. J Card Fail 2007;13(2):137–42.
19. Burkhoff D, Shemer I, Felzen B, et al. Electric currents applied during the refractory period can modulate cardiac contractility in vitro and in vivo. Heart Fail Rev 2001;6(1):27–34.
20. LeWinter MM, Granzier H. Cardiac titin: a multifunctional giant. Circulation 2010;121(19):2137–45.
21. Rastogi S, Mishra S, Zacà V, et al. Effects of chronic therapy with cardiac contractility modulation electrical signals on cytoskeletal proteins and matrix metalloproteinases in dogs with heart failure. Cardiology 2008;110(4):230–7.
22. Ning B, Zhang F, Song X, et al. Cardiac contractility modulation attenuates structural and electrical remodeling in a chronic heart failure rabbit model. J Int Med Res 2020;48(10). 300060520962910.
23. Campbell CM, Kahwash R, Abraham WT. Optimizer Smart in the treatment of moderate-to-severe chronic heart failure. Future Cardiol 2020;16(1):13–25.
24. Butter C, Rastogi S, Minden HH, et al. Cardiac contractility modulation electrical signals improve myocardial gene expression in patients with heart failure. J Am Coll Cardiol 2008;51(18):1784–9.
25. Neelagaru SB, Sanchez JE, Lau SK, et al. Nonexcitatory, cardiac contractility modulation electrical

impulses: feasibility study for advanced heart failure in patients with normal QRS duration. Heart Rhythm 2006;3(10):1140–7.

26. Borggrefe MM, Lawo T, Butter C, et al. Randomized, double blind study of non-excitatory, cardiac contractility modulation electrical impulses for symptomatic heart failure. Eur Heart J 2008;29(8):1019–28.

27. Kadish A, Nademanee K, Volosin K, et al. A randomized controlled trial evaluating the safety and efficacy of cardiac contractility modulation in advanced heart failure. Am Heart J 2011;161(2): 329–37.e1-2.

28. Abraham WT, Kuck KH, Goldsmith RL, et al. A Randomized Controlled Trial to Evaluate the Safety and Efficacy of Cardiac Contractility Modulation. JACC Heart Fail 2018;6(10):874–83.

29. Anker SD, Borggrefe M, Neuser H, et al. Cardiac contractility modulation improves long-term survival and hospitalizations in heart failure with reduced ejection fraction. Eur J Heart Fail 2019;21(9):1103–13.

30. Kuschyk J, Falk P, Demming T, et al. Long-term clinical experience with cardiac contractility modulation therapy delivered by the Optimizer Smart system. Eur J Heart Fail 2021;23(7):1160–9.

31. Wiegn P, Chan R, Jost C, et al. Safety, Performance, and Efficacy of Cardiac Contractility Modulation Delivered by the 2-Lead Optimizer Smart System: The FIX-HF-5C2 Study. Circ Heart Fail 2020;13(4): e006512.

32. Röger S, Schneider R, Rudic B, et al. Cardiac contractility modulation: first experience in heart failure patients with reduced ejection fraction and permanent atrial fibrillation. Europace 2014;16(8): 1205–9.

33. Cleland JG, Daubert JC, Erdmann E, et al. The effect of cardiac resynchronization on morbidity and mortality in heart failure. N Engl J Med 2005;352(15): 1539–49.

34. Kuschyk J, Nägele H, Heinz-Kuck K, et al. Cardiac contractility modulation treatment in patients with symptomatic heart failure despite optimal medical therapy and cardiac resynchronization therapy (CRT). Int J Cardiol 2019;277:173–7.

35. Linde C, Grabowski M, Ponikowski P, et al. Cardiac contractility modulation therapy improves health status in patients with heart failure with preserved ejection fraction: a pilot study (CCM-HFpEF). Eur J Heart Fail 2022. https://doi.org/10.1002/ejhf.2619.

36. Roubertie F, Eschalier R, Zemmoura A, et al. Cardiac Contractility Modulation in a Model of Repaired Tetralogy of Fallot: A Sheep Model. Pediatr Cardiol 2016;37(5):826–33.

37. Contaldi C, De Vivo S, Martucci M, et al. Effects of Cardiac Contractility Modulation Therapy on Right Ventricular Function: An Echocardiographic Study. Appl Sci 2022;7917.

38. Pappone C, Rosanio S, Burkhoff D, et al. Cardiac contractility modulation by electric currents applied during the refractory period in patients with heart failure secondary to ischemic or idiopathic dilated cardiomyopathy. Am J Cardiol 2002;90(12): 1307–13.

Interatrial Shunt Devices

Husam M. Salah, MD[a], Claudia Baratto, MD[b], Dmitry M. Yaranov, MD[c],
Karl-Philipp Rommel, MD[d,e], Satyanarayana Achanta, DVM, PhD, DABT[f],
Sergio Caravita, MD, PhD[b,g], Vinay Kumar Reddy Vasanthu, MBBS[f], Marat Fudim, MD, MHS[h,i],*

KEYWORDS

- Heart failure • Interatrial shunt • HFrEF • HFpEF • Left atrial pressure • Device therapy

KEY POINTS

- Elevated left atrial pressure during exercise is a hallmark of heart failure and is associated with adverse left atrial remodeling, impaired exercise tolerance, and poor long-term outcomes.
- An iatrogenic, pressure-dependent, left-to-right atrial shunt has the potential to decompress the pressure-overloaded left atrium. This decompression may subsequently counteract adverse left atrial remodeling, improve exercise capacity, and decrease heart failure-related poor outcomes.
- Several device-based interatrial shunt approaches have been developed and are currently in various stages of investigations in both heart failure with reduced ejection fraction and heart failure with preserved ejection fraction.
- There is a pressing need for better phenotyping of heart failure to identify those who may benefit the most from interatrial shunt approaches.

INTRODUCTION

Despite several advances in drug therapies for heart failure (HF) over the past decade, HF remains one of the leading causes of hospitalizations with remarkably reduced quality of life and excess morbidity and mortality worldwide.[1,2] In addition, there remain limited pharmacologic options for patients with HF with preserved ejection fraction (HFpEF). Driven by these factors, device-based therapies have emerged as alternative approaches to target structural and biological HF-related abnormalities that may not be amenable to pharmacologic therapies.[3,4]

Elevated left atrial pressure (LAP) at rest and/or during exercise is one of the hallmarks of various phenotypes of HF and is associated with dyspnea, poor exercise capacity, and adverse outcomes (eg, increased mortality).[5–8] Elevated LAP is also associated with adverse left atrial remodeling and dysfunction, pulmonary vascular disease (PVD), and right ventricular dysfunction in both HF with reduced ejection fraction (HFrEF) and HFpEF.[8] The associated adverse left atrial remodeling actively contributes to the progression and clinical course of HF,[9] and several classes of guideline-directed medical therapy indirectly exert their cardiovascular benefits by counteracting adverse left atrial remodeling.[10–12] Based on these observations, it was postulated that a more direct approach to decompress the pressure-overloaded left atrium (eg, by creating an iatrogenic interatrial shunt) may be associated with improved HF-related outcomes. The concept of

Financial Support: none.

[a] Department of Internal Medicine, University of Arkansas for Medical Sciences, Little Rock, AR, USA; [b] Division of Cardiology, Dyspnea and Pulmonary Hypertension Clinic, Ospedale San Luca IRCCS Istituto Auxologico Italiano, Milano, Italy; [c] Baptist Heart Institute, Baptist Memorial Hospital, Memphis, TN, USA; [d] Deptartment of Cardiology, Heart Center at University of Leipzig and Leipzig Heart Institute, Leipzig, Germany; [e] Cardiovacular Research Foundation, New York, NY, USA; [f] Department of Anesthesiology, Duke University School of Medicine, Durham, NC, USA; [g] Department of Management, Information and Production Engineering, University of Bergamo, Dalmine, Province of Bergamo, Italy; [h] Division of Cardiology, Department of Medicine, Duke University, Durham, NC, USA; [i] Duke Clinical Research Institute, Durham, NC, USA

* Corresponding author. Division of Cardiology, Duke University School of Medicine, Duke Clinical Research Institute.

E-mail address: marat.fudim@gmail.com

Heart Failure Clin 20 (2024) 61–69

https://doi.org/10.1016/j.hfc.2023.05.003

an iatrogenic interatrial shunt as a potential therapeutic pathway in patients with HF was further supported by the observation that the presence of concomitant mitral valve stenosis and atrial septal defect (ie, Lutembacher syndrome) is associated with less symptoms and better outcomes when compared with mitral valve stenosis alone.[13,14] Further, surgical closure of atrial septal defects can lead to acute left HF due to an abrupt increase in LAP, necessitating partial reopening of the defect in some cases.[15,16] Early attempts of using the concept of an iatrogenic interatrial shunt were conducted in patients with refractory acute HF under venoarterial extracorporeal membrane oxygenation (VA-ECMO). In such patients, left atrial decompression by creating a left-to-right atrial shunt was associated with improvement in LAP, left-to-right atrial pressure gradient, pulmonary edema, and overall clinical status.[17–20] Subsequently, several device-based approaches were developed to create a permanent controlled left-to-right shunt for left atrial decompression in patients with HF. This review summarizes the current and future landscape of these devices. Conceptually, there are two types of device-based shunts[1]: Shunt is created, and a stent-like structure is left behind (implant-based approach) or[2] shunt is created, and nothing is left behind (implant-free approach).

IMPLANT-BASED APPROACHES
InterAtrial Shunt Device

InterAtrial Shunt Device (IASD, Corvia Medical) is a device-based self-expanding metal stent with a double-disc shape and a central opening of 8 mm that is implanted across the interatrial septum.[3] IASD system is delivered percutaneously via femoral venous access (16 Fr) followed by a standard trans-septal puncture of the interatrial septum and positioning of the device using an over-the-wire technique.[21] IASD placement creates an anatomic communication between the left and right atria, which allows for a pressure-dependent left-to-right flow.[21]

The REDUCE LAP-HF was an open-label, single-arm, phase 1 study that included 68 symptomatic HF patients (despite medical therapy) with left ventricular ejection fraction (LVEF) greater than 40% and pulmonary capillary wedge pressure (PCWP) greater than 15 mm Hg at rest or greater than 25 mm Hg during exercise with the aim to assess the safety and performance of the IASD.[21] The study demonstrated a good safety profile for IASD; no patient experienced periprocedural or major adverse cardiac or cerebrovascular events or needed surgical

intervention for device-related complications at 6 months.[21] At 6 months, 52% of the patients had a reduction in PCWP at rest, and 58% had a reduction in PCWP during exercise.[21] In addition, mean exercise PCWP was significantly lower at 6 months compared with baseline despite increased mean exercise duration.[21] Subsequently, the phase 2 REDUCE LAP-HF I study randomized 44 patients with LVEF $\geq$40%, exercise PCWP $\geq$ 25 mm Hg, and PCWP-right atrial pressure gradient $\geq$5 mm Hg to either IASD implantation or a sham procedure.[22] Compared with sham control, IASD implantation resulted in a greater reduction in PCWP during exercise at 1 month (P = .028) with no periprocedural or major adverse cardiac, cerebrovascular, or renal adverse events in the IASD group at 1-month follow-up (**Fig. 1**).[22] Based on these results, the US Food and Drug Administration granted the IASD system a breakthrough device designation in 2019.[3]

Following that, the phase 3 REDUCE LAP-HF II trial randomized 626 symptomatic HF patients with LVEF $\geq$40%, exercise PCWP $\geq$ 25 mm Hg, and PCWP-right atrial pressure gradient $\geq$5 mm Hg to either IASD implantation or sham procedure.[23] The primary endpoint was a hierarchical composite of cardiovascular mortality or nonfatal ischemic stroke at 12 months, total HF events at 24 months, and change in Kansas City Cardiomyopathy Questionnaire (KCCQ) overall summary score at 12 months.[23] The study showed no difference between the two groups in the primary composite endpoint (win ratio 1.0 [95% CI 0.8–1.2]) or the individual components of the primary composite endpoint. There was also no difference in the composite safety endpoint between the two groups (P = .11).[23] However, prespecified subgroup analyses of the REDUCE LAP-HF II trial demonstrated a differential effect of IASD on HF events based on pulmonary artery systolic pressure at 20 W exercise (pulmonary artery systolic pressure >70 mm Hg was associated with worse outcomes), right atrial volume index (a value > 29.7 mL/m^2 was associated with worse outcomes), and sex (male sex was associated with worse outcomes).[23] As IASD reduces PCWP by pressure-dependent redistributing of blood from the left to the right heart, an increase in pulmonary blood flow (up to 25%) is expected to occur.[24] Although the increase in pulmonary blood flow is associated with favorable outcomes in the short term, a sustained increase in pulmonary blood flow (eg, with renal dialysis access) can be associated with the development of right HF.[25] Driven by these observations, it is expected that creating an atrial shunt in patients with concurrent PVD and elevated LAP

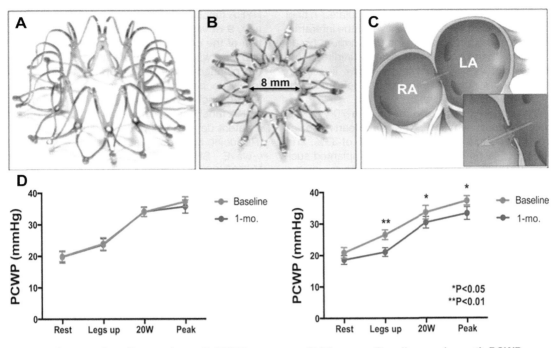

Fig. 1. (*A*, *B*) Different views of the Interatrial Shunt Device (IASD) System. (*C*) The IASD system creates a pressure-dependent left-to-right atrial shunt that decompresses the pressure-overloaded left atrium. (*D*) Changes in pulmonary capillary wedge pressure (PCWP) during exercise hemodynamic testing at 1 month following IASD versus control. ([A-C] Ted Feldman et al., Transcatheter Interatrial Shunt Device for the Treatment of Heart Failure With Preserved Ejection Fraction (REDUCE LAP-HF I [Reduce Elevated Left Atrial Pressure in Patients With Heart Failure]), Circulation. 2018;137:364–375. 15 Nov 2017. https://doi.org/10.1161/CIRCULATIONAHA.117.032094. [D] From Fudim M, Abraham WT, von Bardeleben RS, et al. Device Therapy in Chronic Heart Failure: JACC State-of-the-Art Review. J Am Coll Cardiol. 2021;78(9):931-956.)

would be associated with worse outcomes. Although the REDUCE LAP-HF II trial excluded patients with severe PVD, which was defined as a resting pulmonary vascular resistance (PVR) of greater than 3.5 Wood units (WU); a growing body of evidence suggests that many patients display a more subtle form of PVD that is not identifiable on imaging or invasive testing at rest but becomes apparent during exercise (ie, latent PVD).[26,27] Therefore, a differential effect of IASD on clinical outcomes based on the presence of latent PVD may exist.[28] In a post hoc analysis of the REDUCE LAP-HF II trial, in which the primary outcome was analyzed based on the presence of latent PVD (defined as PVR ≥1.74 WU at peak exercise), IASD implantation was associated with a signal of better outcomes in patients without latent PVD (win ratio 1.31 [95% CI, 1.02, 1.68]) and with worse outcomes in those with latent PVD (win ratio 0.60 [95% CI, 0.42, 0.86]).[28] It remains to be established whether latent PVD is a disease per se or a marker of right heart dysfunction, undermining the ability of these patients to cope with the increased right-sided cardiac flow: latent PVD patients were older, with more atrial fibrillation, more frequently had a pacemaker and presented with more dysfunctional right ventricles with lower cardiac output as well as with larger right atrial volumes than patients without latent PVD.

The RESPONDER-HF (Re-Evaluation of the Corvia Atrial Shunt Device in a Precision Medicine Trial to Determine Efficacy in Mildly Reduced or Preserved Ejection Fraction Heart Failure; NCT05425459) trial is a randomized, sham-controlled, double-blinded trial that aims to evaluate the efficacy and safety of IASD in patients with chronic symptomatic HF, LVEF ≥40%, and hemodynamic evidence of absence of latent PVD (peak exercise PVR < 1.75 WU).

V-Wave Interatrial Shunt

The V-Wave interatrial shunt is a percutaneously implanted (using transfemoral venous access), hourglass-shaped device. The initial design of the V-Wave consisted of an encapsulated nitinol frame that is implanted at the level of the interatrial septum and a trileaflet porcine pericardium tissue valve inside the frame to allow for a unidirectional left-to-right pressure-dependent flow (ie, when the pressure gradient between the left and right atria exceeds 5 mm Hg).

In a first-in-human experience in a 70-year-old patient with ischemic HF, New York Heart Association (NYHA) functional class III, LVEF of 35%, and PCWP of 19 mm Hg, V-Wave was implanted successfully with no complications.[29] At 3 months follow-up, NYHA functional class improved to class II, and PCWP decreased to 8 mm Hg.[29] There was also an improvement in KCCQ score and N-terminal (NT)-pro hormone brain natriuretic peptide (NT-proBNP).[29] In a subsequent single-arm, open-label study of 38 patients (30 patients with HFrEF and 8 patients with HFpEF) with NYHA functional class III–IV despite medical therapy, implantation of the V-Wave system resulted in an improvement in NYHA functional class (60% of the patients improved to class I–II), quality of life in 73% of patients, and 6-min walk distance (mean increase 28 ± 83 m) at 12-month follow-up with a 2.6% rate of the major device- or procedure-related complications during that period.[30] However, late valve-related pannus formation resulting in shunt narrowing/occlusion was observed in up to 50% of the patients at 12-month follow-up.[31] Following this initial experience, a second-generation V-Wave system was developed with valve removal being the most important modification in this generation to improve late device patency (**Fig. 2**).[31]

The second-generation V-Wave was subsequently examined in 10 patients with HF and NYHA functional class III–IV despite medical therapy, 9 of whom underwent successful implantation of the device.[31] Six patients (five with HFrEF and one with HFpEF) were alive and completed the planned 1-year follow-up. At the end of the follow-up period, there was an improvement in NYHA functional class (five patients improved to NYHA functional class I–II) and KCCQ score with a patent device in all patients.[31] The RELIEVE-HF (REducing Lung congestIon Symptoms Using the v-wavE Shunt in adVancEd Heart Failure; NCT03499236) is an ongoing randomized, double-blind study that aims to enroll 605 patients with HF (regardless of LVEF) and NYHA functional class II–IV to examine the safety and efficacy of the second-generation of the V-Wave Interatrial Shunt System. Unlike the shunt size of IASD in the REDUCE LAP-HF II trial (ie, 8 mm), the shunt size of V-Wave in the RELIEVE-HF trial is smaller (ie, 5.1 mm), which may permit less blood flow from left-to-right atria and consequently limit the blood flow into the right ventricle and pulmonary vessels. The relatively less blood flow (compared with IASD) in the right ventricle and pulmonary vessels may subsequently attenuate the differential effect of the shunt based on the presence of latent PVD.

Occlutech Atrial Flow Regulator

The Occlutech atrial flow regulator (AFR) is a percutaneously implanted (using transfemoral venous access), double-disc device with self-expanding nitinol wire mesh that conforms completely to the right septum, creating an interatrial communication with a preselected fixed diameter.[32] The AFR-PRELIEVE was a prospective,

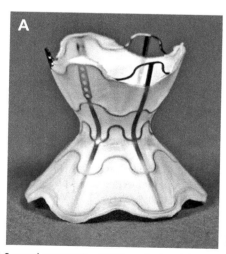
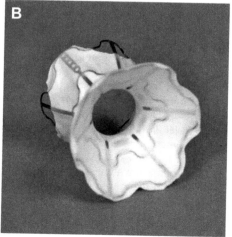

Fig. 2. (*A*) Second-generation V-Wave device. (*B*) View of the valveless lumen of the second-generation V-Wave. (*From* Guimarães L, Bergeron S, Bernier M, et al. Interatrial shunt with the second-generation V-Wave system for patients with advanced chronic heart failure. EuroIntervention. 2020;15(16):1426-1428.)

non-randomized, open-label pilot study that included patients with NYHA functional class III–IV and PCWP ≥15 mm Hg at rest or ≥25 mm Hg at exercise who underwent implantation of the AFR device.[33] In the 3-month results of the AFR-PRELIEVE study with 36 patients (16 patients with HFrEF and 20 patients with HFpEF), the device remained patent in all patients and resulted in improvement in NYHA class, 6-minute walk distance, KCCQ, PCWP, and NT-proBNP.[33] Subsequently, the 1-year results with 53 patients (24 patients with HFrEF and 29 patients with HFpEF) showed consistent results related to efficacy, safety, and device patency,[34] and the 1-year follow-up data from 34 patients (24 patients with HFrEF and 10 patients with HFpEF) demonstrated an observed mortality (3.1/100 patient-years) that was better than the predicted mortality (13.4/100 patient-years) in these patients.[35] The FROST-HF (Flow Regulation by Opening the SepTum in Patients With Heart Failure; a Prospective, Randomized, Sham-controlled, Double-blind, Global Multicenter Study; NCT05136820) is an ongoing randomized, sham-controlled- double-blind trial that aims to enroll 698 patients with chronic symptomatic HF and NYHA functional class II–IV (regardless of LVEF) to examine the efficacy and safety of the AFR with two shunt sizes being examined (6 and 8 mm) and compared with sham.

Transcatheter Atrial Shunt System

The transcatheter atrial shunt system (Edwards Lifesciences) is a percutaneously implanted (using transjugular venous access) device that consists of a bare-nitinol implant edged by four arms (two arms sit on the left atrial wall, and the other two arms lie within the coronary sinus) with an internal shunting diameter of 7 mm.[36] Transcatheter atrial shunt system allows for an atrial-to-coronary sinus shunting, so technically it is not an interatrial shunt.[36] In a first-in-human study, 11 patients (7 with HFpEF and 4 with HFrEF) with symptomatic HF and NYHA functional class III or ambulatory class IV despite medical therapy underwent attempted implantation of the transcatheter atrial shunt system (Edwards Lifesciences). The procedure was successful in eight patients but unsuccessful in the other three patients due to the inability to track the guidewire in the coronary sinus in these patients.[36] During a median follow-up of 201 days, there were no major periprocedural adverse events, and the patients with successful implantation experienced an improvement in NYHA functional class and PCWP with patent devices.[36] The early feasibility ALt FLOW US study (NCT03523416) is an ongoing study that aims to

evaluate the safety, device functionality, and effectiveness of the transcatheter atrial shunt system in 75 patients with symptomatic HF. Although an atrial-to-coronary sinus shunting system may minimize some of the risks associated with interatrial shunting (eg, right-to-left shunting, systemic embolization), its association with other risks (eg, right HF, the effects of volume overload on coronary sinus, and the associated hemodynamic and clinical consequences) remains unclear.

D-Shant Atrium Shunt Device

D-shant atrium shunt device (Wuhan Vickor Medical Technology Co, Ltd) is a percutaneously implanted double disc with a buckle-shaped, nickel-titanium, alloy mesh plug that is implanted in the atrial septum, creating a pressure-dependent left-to-right shunt.[37] In a retrospective study including six patients with NYHA functional class II–IV HF, the D-shant atrium shunt device was associated with a significant reduction in left ventricular diameter and volume, functional mitral regurgitation, PCWP, and mean LAP (**Fig. 3**).[37]

IMPLANT-FREE APPROACHES
Septal Cutting Balloon

The septal-cutting balloon approach is used to create a septal defect with pressure-dependent left-to-right atrial shunting.[38] The use of this approach was documented in a case report of a 58-year-old female patient with refractory NYHA functional class III and severe postcapillary pulmonary hypertension (mean pulmonary arterial pressure: 49 mm Hg; PCWP: 29 mm Hg; right atrial pressure: 8 mm Hg) secondary to HFpEF.[38] Under biplane transesophageal modality guidance, a transseptal puncture was performed in the mid-fossa ovalis using a radiofrequency transseptal needle. A cutting balloon was then positioned in the hole, inflated and deflated every 5 seconds, and rotated clockwise every 60 seconds. Following the procedure, pulmonary arterial pressure and PCWP improved significantly.[38] NYHA functional class improved to class 2 within a month and remained the same at 6 months follow-up. The shunt remained patent and unidirectional during follow-ups.[38]

Alleviant System

The Alleviant System creates an implant-free interatrial shunt. Following transseptal puncture, the Alleviant System is used to excise a segment of the interatrial septum with a target shunt diameter of 7 mm via 0.5-second radiofrequency energy under fluoroscopic and echocardiographic guidance (**Fig. 4**).[39] Preliminary results from HFpEF studies

	IASD	V-Wave	Occlutech AFR	Transcatheter atrial shunt system (atrial-to-coronary sinus)	D-shant
	(device image)	(device image)	(device image)	(device image)	(device image)
Heart failure phenotype	HFpEF	HFrEF and HFpEF	HFrEF and HFpEF	HFrEF and HFpEF	HFrEF and HFpEF
PCWP	Rest → / Exercise ↓	Rest − / Exercise ?	Rest ↓ / Exercise ?	Rest ↓ / Exercise ?	Rest ↓ / Exercise ?
NYHA	↓	↓	↓	↓	↓
6MWD	?	−	↑	↑	↑

Fig. 3. Clinical effects of implant-based interatrial shunt devices based on the currently available evidence (the level of evidence for the clinical effects of each device varies). 6MWD, 6-min walk distance; HFpEF, heart failure with preserved ejection fraction; HFrEF; heart failure with reduced ejection fraction; NYHA, New York Heart Association; PCWP, pulmonary capillary wedge pressure. (*Created with* BioRender.com.)

(ALLEVIATE-HF-1 and ALLEVIATE-HF-2) and a dedicated HFrEF study with a total of 30 patients showed successful procedures with no device-related adverse events in all patients.[39] The Alleviant System decreased the mean peak exercise PCWP and increased the overall KCCQ score.[39] At 6 months, shunt size remained stable, and there was a decrease in left atrial diameter in patients with HFpEF (−2.4 mm; $P = .031$).[39] The pivotal ALLAY HF trial has been kicked off in 2023 with a trial population similar to RESPONDER HF (NCT NCT05685303).

Atrial Septostomy Device (NoYA System)

Atrial septostomy device (NoYA system, NoYA MedTech, Hangzhou, China) is a percutaneous radiofrequency ablation-based interatrial shunting therapy that creates an artificial atrial septal defect with no implants.[40] The system consists of a self-expanded flowerlike nitinol stent that is connected to a radiofrequency generator. After the completion of radiofrequency ablation, the device is completely removed, leaving nothing but the artificial atrial septal defect.[40] The first-in-human RAISE trial included 10 patients with HFpEF who underwent interatrial shunting therapy.[40] At 6 months of follow-up, no major safety events were observed, and continuous shunting was still observed in seven patients by the end of the follow-up period.[40] NoYA system resulted in a significant improvement in the clinical status with the reduction in NT-proBNP, increase in 6-minute walk distance, and improvement in NYHA functional class.[40] The NoYA RAISE Trial II (A Prospective, Multi-center and Objective Performance Criteria Study to Evaluate the Effectiveness and Safety of NoYA Radiofrequency Interatrial Shunt System for the Treatment of Chronic Heart Failure With Elevated Left Atrial Pressure; NCT05375110)

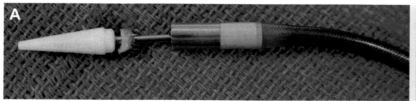
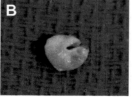

Fig. 4. The atrial septostomy device (Alleviant). (*A*) Septal crossing and radiofrequency ablation of the septum. (*B*) Septal tissue removed via radiofrequency ablation. (*Courtesy of* Alleviant, Austin, TX, with permission.)

is an ongoing, single-arm, open-label, prospective study that aims to enroll 120 patients with chronic symptomatic HF (NYHA functional class II–IV), elevated LAP, and LVEF ≥15% to examine the efficacy and safety of the NoYA Radiofrequency Interatrial Shunt System for the treatment of chronic HF with elevated LAP.

InterShunt PAS-C System

InterShunt percutaneous atrial shunt catheter (PAS-C) is another implant-free interatrial shunt system that is delivered percutaneously via transfemoral venous access and deployed in the left atrium following transseptal crossing under fluoroscopic and echocardiographic guidance.[41,42] Following deployment in the left atrium, the InterShunt PAS-C system is used to capture, cut, and remove tissue from the interatrial septum based on prescribed surface area and shape.[41] In preliminary results of a feasibility study including eight patients with HF and NYHA functional class II–IV, deployment of the InterShunt PAS-C system was successful in all patients with no device-related adverse events, and the left-to-right shunt remained patent at 1-month follow-up.[41] In addition, the mean peak exercise PCWP decreased by 6 mm Hg and the mean NT-proBNP decreased by 405.6 pg/mL.[41] The EASE HF (Evaluation of an Implant Free Interatrial Shunt to Improve Heart Failure; NCT05403372) study is still ongoing and aims to provide more information related to the safety and efficacy of the InterShunt PAS-C system.

SUMMARY AND FUTURE DIRECTIONS

Elevated LAP is a driving mechanism for several of the manifestations of HF and is associated with poor outcomes in both HFrEF and HFpEF. Several implant-based and non-implant-based device therapies were developed to create pressure-dependent, left-to-right atrial shunting systems to decompress the pressure-overloaded left atrium in HF (see **Fig. 3**). Although phase 1 and phase 2 studies of various atrial shunting systems have generally shown favorable safety profiles and encouraging signals of clinical benefits, the only phase 3 clinical trial (ie, REDUCE LAP-HF II) failed to show a reduction in HF events or health status improvement in the overall population of patients with LVEF of ≥40%. However, a post hoc analysis of the REDUCE LAP-HF II trial uncovered possible benefits in those without latent PVD and revealed a signal of harm in those with latent PVD, suggesting a differential effect of interatrial shunting on clinical outcomes based on the presence of latent PVD. This observation informs future and ongoing clinical trials in the field and underscores the importance of better phenotyping of HF to identify those who would benefit the most from device-based therapies and help exclude those who may experience harm.

OPEN QUESTIONS

Future investigations will need to determine the following critical questions.

- Identify the ideal patient population and confirm whether latent PVD is the key differentiator of response.
- Resolve the apparent discrepancy between trial populations, which differ significantly in proposed key variables to predict benefit and risk from interatrial shunting, such as right ventricular dysfunction and PVD (aka RESPONDER HF/ALLAY HF vs RELEASE HF).
- Although a direct comparison of implant-based and implant-free shunt approaches is unlikely to happen, the critical review of benefits of each approach is needed. Considerations should include the evaluation of the limitations of an implant-based approach and potential limitations it provides to procedures requiring interatrial crossing (pulmonary vein isolation, atrial appendage closures, mitraclip, and so forth.). Additional considerations need to be given to the impact of implant-based approaches on the immobilization of the interatrial septum. Because the interatrial septum is contributing to the atrial reservoir function, implant-free approaches might have distinct benefit by avoiding a restriction of the septum.
- The question of the correct size of the shunt remains unresolved. It is very likely that one size does not fit all, and future phenotyping approaches will have to match shunt size to HF physiology (and take the longitudinal nature of progressive right ventricular and left ventricular failure into consideration).
- Although patency has so far not been an issue for the new-generation shunts (whether implant-based or implant-free), future long-term safety outcomes are needed, particularly for the implant-free devices given that there are less cases documented to date for those technologies.

CLINICS CARE POINTS

- Elevated left atrial pressure is a poor prognostic factor in patients with heart failure (HF).

- Current evidence does not support the use of interatrial shunts to decompress the left atrium in patients with HF with reduced ejection fraction or HF with preserved ejection fraction (HFpEF). However, there is a signal of possible benefits of interatrial shunts in patients with HFpEF and hemodynamic evidence of the absence of latent pulmonary vascular disease (ie, peak exercise pulmonary vascular resistance < 1.75 WU).

DISCLOSURES

Dr M. Fudim was supported by the American Heart Association, United States (20IPA35310955), Doris Duke, United States, Bayer, United States, Bodyport, United States, and Verily. He receives consulting fees from Abbott, Ajax, Alio Health, Alleviant, Audicor, AxonTherapies, Bayer, Bodyguide, Bodyport, Boston Scientific, Broadview, Cadence, Cardionomics, Coridea, CVRx, Daxor, Deerfield Catalyst, Edwards LifeSciences, EKO, Feldschuh Foundation, Fire1, Galvani, Gradient, Hatteras, Impulse Dynamics, Intershunt, Medtronic, Merck, NIMedical, NovoNordisk, NucleusRx, NXT Biomedical, Pharmacosmos, PreHealth, ReCor, Shifamed, Splendo, Sumacor, SyMap, Verily, Vironix, Viscardia, and Zoll. Dr D.M. Yaranov is supported by research grant from Daxor and Nuwelis, United States. Dr K-P. Rommel is supported by a research grant from the Else-Kröner-Fresenius-Stiftung, United States, Bad Homburg, United States, Germany. Dr S. Achanta is supported by research grants from the NIEHS-NIH CounterACT program, United States (1R01-ES034387–01; 5R21-ES030331–02; 5R21-ES033020–02; 5U01-ES030672–03) and VisCardia, Inc. All other authors declare no disclosures.

REFERENCES

1. Salah HM, Minhas AMK, Khan MS, et al. Trends in hospitalizations for heart failure, acute myocardial infarction, and stroke in the United States from 2004 to 2018. Am Heart J 2022;243:103–9.
2. Salah HM, Minhas AMK, Khan MS, et al. Causes of hospitalization in the USA between 2005 and 2018. Eur Heart J Open 2021;1:oeab001.
3. Fudim M, Abraham WT, von Bardeleben RS, et al. Device Therapy in Chronic Heart Failure: JACC State-of-the-Art Review. J Am Coll Cardiol 2021;78:931–56.
4. Salah HM, Levin AP, Fudim M. Device Therapy for Heart Failure with Preserved Ejection Fraction. Cardiol Clin 2022;40:507–15.
5. Dorfs S, Zeh W, Hochholzer W, et al. Pulmonary capillary wedge pressure during exercise and long-term mortality in patients with suspected heart failure with preserved ejection fraction. Eur Heart J 2014;35:3103–12.
6. Eisman AS, Shah RV, Dhakal BP, et al. Pulmonary Capillary Wedge Pressure Patterns During Exercise Predict Exercise Capacity and Incident Heart Failure. Circulation: Heart Fail 2018;11:e004750.
7. Ahlgrim C, Kocher S, Minners J, et al. Pulmonary Capillary Wedge Pressure during Exercise Is Prognostic for Long-Term Survival in Patients with Symptomatic Heart Failure. J Clin Med 2022;11.
8. Obokata M, Olson TP, Reddy YNV, et al. Haemodynamics, dyspnoea, and pulmonary reserve in heart failure with preserved ejection fraction. Eur Heart J 2018;39:2810–21.
9. Inciardi RM, Bonelli A, Biering-Sorensen T, et al. Left atrial disease and left atrial reverse remodelling across different stages of heart failure development and progression: a new target for prevention and treatment. Eur J Heart Fail 2022;24:959–75.
10. Bode D, Semmler L, Wakula P, et al. Dual SGLT-1 and SGLT-2 inhibition improves left atrial dysfunction in HFpEF. Cardiovasc Diabetol 2021;20:7.
11. Salah HM, Verma S, Santos-Gallego CG, et al. Sodium-Glucose Cotransporter 2 Inhibitors and Cardiac Remodeling. Journal of Cardiovascular Translational Research 2022;15:944–56.
12. Sun Y, Song S, Zhang Y, et al. Effect of angiotensin receptor neprilysin inhibitors on left atrial remodeling and prognosis in heart failure. ESC Heart Fail 2022;9:667–75.
13. Jørgensen TH, Søndergaard L. Transcatheter Implantation of Interatrial Shunt Devices to Lower Left Atrial Pressure in Heart Failure. Int J Heart Fail 2022;4:12–23.
14. Lutembacher R. De la sténose mitrale avec communication interauriculaire. Arch Mal Coeur 1916;9:237–60.
15. Beyer J. Atrial Septal Defect: Acute Left Heart Failure After Surgical Closure. Ann Thorac Surg 1978;25:36–43.
16. Ewert P, Berger F, Nagdyman N, et al. Masked left ventricular restriction in elderly patients with atrial septal defects: A contraindication for closure? Cathet Cardiovasc Interv 2001;52:177–80.
17. Seib PM, Faulkner SC, Erickson CC, et al. Blade and balloon atrial septostomy for left heart decompression in patients with severe ventricular dysfunction on extracorporeal membrane oxygenation. Cathet Cardiovasc Interv 1999;46:179–86.
18. Johnston TA, Jaggers J, McGovern JJ, et al. Bedside transseptal balloon dilation atrial septostomy for decompression of the left heart during extracorporeal membrane oxygenation. Cathet Cardiovasc Interv 1999;46:197–9.

19. Aiyagari RM, Rocchini AP, Remenapp RT, et al. Decompression of the left atrium during extracorporeal membrane oxygenation using a transseptal cannula incorporated into the circuit. Crit Care Med 2006;34:2603–6.

20. Baruteau A-E, Barnetche T, Morin L, et al. Percutaneous balloon atrial septostomy on top of venoarterial extracorporeal membrane oxygenation results in safe and effective left heart decompression. European Heart Journal Acute Cardiovascular Care 2018;7:70–9.

21. Hasenfuß G, Hayward C, Burkhoff D, et al. A transcatheter intracardiac shunt device for heart failure with preserved ejection fraction (REDUCE LAP-HF): a multicentre, open-label, single-arm, phase 1 trial. Lancet 2016;387:1298–304.

22. Feldman T, Mauri L, Kahwash R, et al. Transcatheter Interatrial Shunt Device for the Treatment of Heart Failure With Preserved Ejection Fraction (REDUCE LAP-HF I [Reduce Elevated Left Atrial Pressure in Patients With Heart Failure]). Circulation 2018;137:364–75.

23. Shah SJ, Borlaug BA, Chung ES, et al. Atrial shunt device for heart failure with preserved and mildly reduced ejection fraction (REDUCE LAP-HF II): a randomised, multicentre, blinded, sham-controlled trial. Lancet 2022;399:1130–40.

24. Obokata M, Reddy YNV, Shah SJ, et al. Effects of Interatrial Shunt on Pulmonary Vascular Function in Heart Failure With Preserved Ejection Fraction. J Am Coll Cardiol 2019;74:2539–50.

25. Reddy YNV, Obokata M, Dean PG, et al. Long-term cardiovascular changes following creation of arteriovenous fistula in patients with end stage renal disease. Eur Heart J 2017;38:1913–23.

26. Borlaug BA, Kane GC, Melenovsky V, et al. Abnormal right ventricular-pulmonary artery coupling with exercise in heart failure with preserved ejection fraction. Eur Heart J 2016;37:3293–302.

27. Ho JE, Zern EK, Lau ES, et al. Exercise Pulmonary Hypertension Predicts Clinical Outcomes in Patients With Dyspnea on Effort. J Am Coll Cardiol 2020;75:17–26.

28. Borlaug BA, Blair J, Bergmann MW, et al. Latent Pulmonary Vascular Disease May Alter the Response to Therapeutic Atrial Shunt Device in Heart Failure. Circulation 2022;145:1592–604.

29. Amat-Santos IJ, Bergeron S, Bernier M, et al. Left atrial decompression through unidirectional left-to-right interatrial shunt for the treatment of left heart failure: first-in-man experience with the V-Wave device. EuroIntervention 2015;10:1127–31.

30. Rodés-Cabau J, Bernier M, Amat-Santos IJ, et al. Interatrial Shunting for Heart Failure: Early and Late Results From the First-in-Human Experience With the V-Wave System. JACC Cardiovasc Interv 2018;11:2300–10.

31. Guimarães L, Bergeron S, Bernier M, et al. Interatrial shunt with the second-generation V-Wave system for patients with advanced chronic heart failure. EuroIntervention 2020;15:1426–8.

32. Rajeshkumar R, Pavithran S, Sivakumar K, et al. Atrial septostomy with a predefined diameter using a novel Occlutech atrial flow regulator improves symptoms and cardiac index in patients with severe pulmonary arterial hypertension. Cathet Cardiovasc Interv 2017;90:1145–53.

33. Paitazoglou C, Özdemir R, Pfister R, et al. The AFR-PRELIEVE trial: a prospective, non-randomised, pilot study to assess the Atrial Flow Regulator (AFR) in heart failure patients with either preserved or reduced ejection fraction. EuroIntervention 2019;15:403–10.

34. Paitazoglou C, Bergmann MW, Özdemir R, et al. One-year results of the first-in-man study investigating the Atrial Flow Regulator for left atrial shunting in symptomatic heart failure patients: the PRELIEVE study. Eur J Heart Fail 2021;23:800–10.

35. Bakhshaliyev N, Çelikkale İ, Enhoş A, et al. Impact of atrial flow regulator (AFR) implantation on 12-month mortality in heart failure. Herz 2022;47:366–73.

36. Simard T, Labinaz M, Zahr F, et al. Percutaneous Atriotomy for Levoatrial-to-Coronary Sinus Shunting in Symptomatic Heart Failure: First-in-Human Experience. JACC Cardiovasc Interv 2020;13:1236–47.

37. Shang X, Liu M, Zhong Y, et al. Clinical study on the treatment of chronic heart failure with a novel D-shant atrium shunt device. ESC Heart Fail 2022;9:1713–20.

38. Bauer F, Besnier E, Aludaat C, et al. Left atrial unloading with an 8 mm septal cutting balloon to treat postcapillary pulmonary hypertension: a case report. ESC Heart Fail 2022;9:782–5.

39. Barker CM, Wilkins G, Wilkins B, et al. LB-6 | No-implant Interatrial Shunt for Heart Failure: Multicenter Clinical Outcomes. Journal of the Society for Cardiovascular Angiography & Interventions 2022;1.

40. Sun W, Zou H, Yong Y, et al. The RAISE Trial: A Novel Device and First-in-Man Trial. Circulation: Heart Fail 2022;15:e008362.

41. Vardi G, Meece R, Shaburishvili T, et al. TCT-343 Evaluation of an Implant Free Interatrial Shunt to Improve Heart Failure: EASE HF. J Am Coll Cardiol 2022;80:B139.

42. Sivakumar K, Rohitraj GR, Rajendran M, et al. Study of the effect of Occlutech Atrial Flow Regulator on symptoms, hemodynamics, and echocardiographic parameters in advanced pulmonary arterial hypertension. Pulm Circ 2021;11. 2045894021989966.

Preload Reduction Therapies in Heart Failure

Muhammad Shahzeb Khan, MBBS[a], Anousheh Awais Paracha, MBBS[b,1], Jan Biegus, MD[c], Rafael de la Espriella, MD[d], Julio Núñez, MD[d,e,f], Carlos G. Santos-Gallego, MD[g,h], Dmitry Yaranov, MD[i], Marat Fudim, MD, MHS[a,j],*

KEYWORDS

- Heart failure • Congestion • Preload • Stressed blood volume • Unstressed blood volume

KEY POINTS

- The recruitment of preload is a physiological response to a stressed state such as exercise but in heart failure an increase in preload leads to an excessive increase in intracardiac pressures.
- The reduction of preload can be achieved via number of pharmacological and nonpharmacological interventions.
- Nonpharmacological interventions seek to reduce inflow to the heart or increase splanchnic vascular blood pooling.

INTRODUCTION

Preload reserve represents a central concept in the understanding of the cardiovascular system physiology. This refers to the ability to increase cardiac output (CO) via an augmented venous return in order to meet the varying metabolic demands of the body. Veins serve not only to return the blood to the heart but also to act as functional reservoirs of blood containing around 70% of the total blood volume (TBV). In contrast, only 30% of the TBV is contained within arteries.[1,2] Additionally, the TBV of the body is functionally divided into 2 parts: UBV and SBV (TBV = UBV [unstressed blood volume] + SBV [stressed blood volume]), respectively.[1,3] The UBV is the volume of blood needed to fill a vessel till the wall stress and intravascular pressure increase just above 0 mm Hg, whereas the SBV is the volume in the vessel in addition to the UBV determining the stress and intravascular pressure thereby altering the CO.[4]

Despite the importance of preload reserve in healthy patients, in patients with acute and chronic heart failure (HF), the decreased venous capacitance causes a concomitant increase in filling pressures at rest and with exercise, which is associated with worse HF signs and symptoms as well as outcomes. Therefore, the recruitment of preload to improve CO may exacerbate exercise intolerance and precipitate HF decompensation.[5] Accordingly, recent studies have focused on various interventions for cardiac preload reduction in patients with HF and important advances have been made in this area. This may be achieved via unloading of the heart with an increase in UBV and decrease in SBV through either splanchnic nerve modulation (SNM) or pharmacological interventions. On the contrary, the heart may be unloaded without changing the UBV or SBV that is, through a superior vena cava (SVC) or inferior vena cava (IVC) inflow block. In this review, we

[a] Division of Cardiology, Department of Medicine, Duke University, Durham, NC, USA; [b] Department of Medicine, Dow University of Health Sciences, Karachi, Pakistan; [c] Institute of Heart Diseases, Wroclaw Medical University, Poland; [d] Cardiology Department, Hospital Clínico Universitario de Valencia, Fundación de Investigación INCLIVA, Valencia, Spain; [e] Department of Medicine, University of Valencia, Valencia, Spain; [f] CIBER Cardiovascular, Madrid, Spain; [g] Cardiology Department, Mount Sinai Hospital, NYC; [h] Cardiovascular Institute, Icahn School of Medicine at Mount Sinai, NYC; [i] Baptist Memorial Healthcare, Memphis, TN, USA; [j] Duke Clinical Research Institute, Durham, NC, USA

[1] Primary coauthor.
* Corresponding author.
E-mail address: marat.fudim@duke.edu

Heart Failure Clin 20 (2024) 71–81
https://doi.org/10.1016/j.hfc.2023.05.004
1551-7136/24/© 2023 Elsevier Inc. All rights reserved.

aim to provide a mechanistic overview of pharmacological interventions, SNM, and novel cardiac preload reduction therapies aimed at management of HF while discussing emerging evidence to help guide future clinical use (**Fig. 1**).

PRELOAD REDUCTION THERAPIES: PHARMACOLOGICAL INTERVENTIONS

Studies have shown an integral role of pharmacological therapies in preload reduction via unloading of the heart with an increase in UBV and decrease in SBV. Research in both animals and humans show the effects of vasodilator drugs such as hydralazine, enalaprilat, and nitroglycerin on the SBV. Wang and colleagues[6] studied the differential effects of these drugs by experimental induction of acute ischemic HF in 19 splenectomized dogs, which resulted in a 14% splanchnic venoconstriction, a leftward shift of the pressure–volume curve, and a significant increase in the left-ventricular end-diastolic pressure (LVEDP; **Table 1**). Data show that the administration of nitroglycerin and enalaprilat (not hydralazine) contributed to splanchnic venodilation and reduction of LVEDP, thereby modulating changes in left ventricular preload. Similarly, Okamoto and colleagues[7] used a

radionuclide method to assess the splanchnic capacitance (pressure–volume relationship) and compliance before and after the usage of 0.6 mg sublingual nitroglycerin. There was a significant increase in splanchnic capacitance and compliance thereby reducing cardiac filling pressures. Sarma and colleagues[8] evaluated the acute reductions in pulmonary capillary wedge pressure (PCWP) in 30 patients with HFpEF with and without nitroglycerin. Results showed that administration of nitroglycerin caused a graded decrease in PCWP at rest, 20 W, and peak exercise; however, these acute reductions in PCWP did not improve functional/exercise capacity. This study was limited due to the usage of a systemic vasodilator. Moreover, earlier data show that isosorbide mononitrate does not improve outcomes in patients with HFpEF.[9] On the contrary, it must be noted that the impacts of preload reduction on long-term functional capacity are yet to be determined, and it is expected that various phenotypes of HF/HFpEF will have a differential response to significant preload reduction. The role of phenotypes on therapies that reduce left atrial preload by shunting blood from the left atrium to right atrium has been recently demonstrated in the REDUCE-LAP II trial. Higher pulmonary vascular resistance

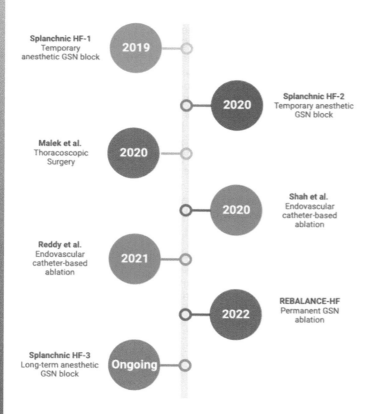

Fig. 1. Targets of various interventions for cardiac preload reduction.

Table 1
Relative hemodynamic changes produced by acute heart failure, enalaprilat, hydralazine, and nitroglycerin

	Control	Acute Heart Failure	Hydralazine	Enalaprilat	Nitroglycerin
Acute Heart Failure (n = 19)					
CO, L/min	3.83 ± 0.9	1.87 ± 0.6	-	-	-
SVR, mm Hg · min/L	31.6 ± 4.9	54.5 ± 6.6	-	-	-
PVP, mm Hg	6.6 ± 0.7	7.1 ± 0.8	-	-	-
SVV, %	100	86 ± 2	-	-	-
LVEDP, mm Hg	6.2 ± 0.4	21.4 ± 1.3			
Enalaprilat (n = 7)					
CO, L/min	4.3 ± 0.5	2.4 ± 0.3	-	2.6 ± 0.2	-
SVR, mm Hg · min/L	27.9 ± 3	45.1 ± 4.3	-	32.2 ± 3.3	-
PVP, mm Hg	7.2 ± 0.9	7.7 ± 0.6	-	7.0 ± 0.5	-
SVV, %	100	85 ± 3	-	96 ± 3	-
LVEDP, mm Hg	7.2 ± 0.4	21.1 ± 1.3	-	15.8 ± 1.3	-
Hydralazine (n = 6)					
CO, L/min	3.7 ± 0.8	1.5 ± 0.5	2.2 ± 0.6	-	-
SVR, mm Hg · min/L	30.3 ± 4.1	53.7 ± 5.9	29.4 ± 3.3	-	-
PVP, mm Hg	6.5 ± 1.0	7.1 ± 0.7	6.2 ± 0.8	-	-
SVV, %	100	86 ± 2	88 ± 3	-	-
LVEDP, mm Hg	6.3 ± 0.5	20.4 ± 1.8	17.8 ± 1.9	-	-
Nitroglycerin (n = 6)					
CO, L/min	3.5 ± 0.7	1.7 ± 0.5	-	-	1.9 ± 0.5
SVR, mm Hg min/L	36.5 ± 2.4	64.6 ± 3.6	-	-	52.5 ± 1.9
PVP, mm Hg	6.2 ± 0.8	6.4 ± 1.2	-	-	5.2 ± 0.7
SVV, %	100	86 ± 2	-	-	113 ± 3
LVEDP, mm Hg	5.0 ± 0.3	22.7 ± 0.9	-	-	13.1 ± 0.4

Values are mean ± SD.
Abbreviations: CO, cardiac output; PVP, mean portal vein pressure; SVR, systemic vascular resistance; SVV, splanchnic vascular volume.

and other surrogates of right-sided dysfunction were found to have a worse outcome with interatrial shunting.[10,11]

Recent analyses have focused on assessing the effects of pharmacological interventions on the estimated stressed blood volume (eSBV). This is due to the technical limitations in measuring the actual SBV through methods that, for example, induce a temporary circulatory arrest.[4] Therefore, this quantity is estimated using computer simulation models that use heart rate, CO, PCWP, central venous pressure (CVP), pulmonary arterial pressure (PAP), left ventricular ejection fraction (LVEF), and systolic and diastolic systemic arterial pressures. Moreover, eSBV values are measured as milliliter per 70 kg body weight due to the variation in patient sizes. In recent studies, focus has shifted toward the impact of different pharmacological therapies on eSBV. Kaye and colleagues[12] studied the effects of milrinone on filling pressures

at rest and during exercise in 10 patients with HFpEF. Results showed a reduction in eSBV from 1539 to 1066 mL. In another investigation, Brener and colleagues[13] measured the effects of a weekly infusion of levosimendan in patients with HFpEF and pulmonary hypertension. Levosimendan reduced the resting SBV from 2750 to 2449 mL. Similarly, Omar and colleagues[14] investigated the effect of empagliflozin, a sodium-glucose cotransporter-2 inhibitor on eSBV in patients with HF with reduced ejection fraction (HFrEF). Administration of 10 mg empagliflozin showed a significant reduction in eSBV of ~200 mL (**Table 2**). Finally, Sorimachi and colleagues[15] compared the eSBV in obese patients with HFpEF versus nonobese patients with HFpEF. Invasive hemodynamic testing showed that eSBV was significantly higher in obese versus nonobese HFpEF patients (**Table 3**). Therefore, these findings show that a reduction in SBV is

Table 2
Baseline characteristics and measurement of stressed blood volume preintervention and postintervention

Study Title	Number of Participants (N)	Primary Outcome	Age (Years)	Intervention	BMI (kg/m²)	LVEF (%)	Resting SBV Preintervention (mL)	Resting SBV Postintervention (mL)	Preintervention SBV at Peak Load	Postintervention SBV at Peak Load (mL)
Kaye et al,[13] 2020	10	Left ventricular end-systolic, end-diastolic pressure–volume relations, stressed blood volume, heart rate, and arterial mechanics	68 ± 2	Milrinone	31 ± 1	64 ± 2	1539	1066	-	-
Brener et al,[14] 2021	35	Mean pulmonary capillary wedge pressure at rest and during exercise	68 ± 9	Levosimendan	34 ± 8	58 ± 8	2750	2449*	-/-	-
Fudim et al,[35] 1995	14	Exercise capacity measured by peak oxygen uptake, mean PAP, and pulmonary capillary wedge pressure	58 ± 13	Splanchnic nerve blockade	31 ± 16	21 ± 12	2664 ± 488	2132 ± 570	3243 ± 352	2662 ± 656
Okamoto et al,[7] 2021	85	Effect of sublingual nitroglycerin (SL NTG) for increasing splanchnic capacitance and compliance	37 ± 44	Nitroglycerin	31 ± 38	-	100 ± 1.81 *	104.6 ± 8.81*	-	-
Omar et al,[15] 2021	35	Change in estimated SBV after 12 wk of empagliflozin treatment	59 ± 8	Empaglifozin	29 ± 6	-	1697 ± 312	1601 ± 337	3269 ± 486	3105 ± 509

Table 3
Baseline characteristics and distribution of blood volume at rest and during exercise

	HFpEF (n = 62)	HFrEF (n = 14)
Age (years)	68 ± 12	58 ± 13
BMI (kg/m²)	33.3 ± 6.9	31 ± 16
LVEF (%)	61 ± 6	21 ± 12
Hypertension, n (%)	47 (76)	4 (29)
Atrial fibrillation, n (%)	21 (34)	7 (50)
Diabetes mellitus, n (%)	14 (23)	4 (29)
Creatinine (mg/dL)	1.0 ± 0.4	1.2 ± 0.4
Beta blockers, n (%)	29 (47)	14 (100)
ACE-I/ARB	20 (32)	10 (71)
Baseline stressed volume (mL)	2494 ± 3162	2664 ± 488
20W stressed volume (mL)	3504 ± 2764	3260 ± 362
Peak stressed volume (mL)	3795 ± 3610	3243 ± 352

Values are mean ± SD or n (%).
Abbreviations: ACE-I, angiotensin-converting enzyme inhibitor; ARB, angiotensin receptor blocker; BMI, body mass index; HFpEF, heart failure with preserved ejection fraction; HFrEF, heart failure with reduced ejection fraction.
Data from Refs.[12,16]

associated with improved resting and exercise hemodynamics in patients with predominantly left-sided HF.

THE SPLANCHNIC COMPARTMENT

The splanchnic circulation is responsible for supplying blood to the stomach, spleen, liver, pancreas, small intestine, and large intestine. This blood flow is modifiable according to the changing needs of the body and is controlled by multiple intrinsic and extrinsic factors. The bilateral sympathetic ganglia provide fibers to the celiac plexus by giving rise to the greater, lesser, and least thoracic splanchnic nerves.[16,17] Accordingly, the blood vessels in this compartment are innervated by the sympathetic nervous system, which alters the capacitance of the splanchnic venous circulation through the greater splanchnic nerve (GSN).[18] This results in venoconstriction and the translocation of blood from the splanchnic bed to the central circulation, that is, from UBV to SBV. Because the splanchnic vascular compartment contains most of the intravascular blood volume, it serves as the major source of vascular capacitance in both animals and humans.[1,19–23] The translocation of blood from the splanchnic to the central circulation leads to increased preload and CO.[3,24,25]

Evidence suggests that the hemodynamic disturbances and exercise intolerance in HF are attributable to the neurohormonal-mediated reduction in vascular capacitance.[3,26] Recent evidence shows that stimulation of the splanchnic nerve causes the translocation of ~80% of the splanchnic volume (20% of the TBV), thereby increasing the actively circulating blood volume and CO.[21,27,28] This concept assumes that in a healthy person once the CO needs to be increased (ie, during exercise) not only a heart rate and stroke volume increase but also actively circulating blood volume needs to be augmented, which allows the lower velocity of arterial flow to maintain the given CO. However, if the cardiovascular system (for any reason) is not able to cope with the augmented preload adequately, it leads to dramatic increase in intracardiac pressures and SBV. Studies in both animals and humans have corroborated these findings.

To further clarify the role of SBV in intracardiac pressures and CO, Kaye and colleagues studied the rest and exercise hemodynamics in 60 patients with HFpEF. Results showed that eSBV was a major contributor to increased cardiac filling pressures (CVP and PCWP) while there was no significant increase in CO.[12,29] Therefore, the role of splanchnic nerve stimulation is integral in cardiac preload modulation.

Bapna and colleagues[30] explored the effectiveness of an implantable cuff system on the GSN in 5 healthy canines and its effect on circulation. Stimulation of the right GSN increased mean arterial blood pressure by 36.9 mm Hg ± 13.4 ($P < .0001$), mean PAP by 6.3 mm Hg ± 2.0 ($P < .0001$), and CVP by 6.9 mm Hg ± 1.7 ($P < .0001$). A case series of 5 patients with pancreatic cancer has recently substantiated these findings. Investigators used irreversible electroporation to evaluate the hemodynamic effects of splanchnic nerve stimulation in humans. Results showed an increase in CO from 3.6 to 6.4 L/min and CVP from 7.2 to 13.6 mm Hg. However, this analysis was limited because redistribution was not evaluated directly but rather indirectly via pressure raises. In addition, there was no neurohormonal testing.[31]

The hemodynamic effects of GSN stimulation in a patient with HFpEF and atrial fibrillation were studied by stimulating the splanchnic nerves for 40 seconds. GSN stimulation resulted in an increase in mean CVP from 6 to 8 mm Hg, mean left atrial pressure from 7 to 14 mm Hg, arterial blood pressure from 85/45 mm Hg to 123/75 mm Hg, and mean PAP from 14 to 21 mm Hg. In addition, intracardiac and central vascular pressures continued to increase after termination of SNM.[32]

DEVICE-BASED PRELOAD REDUCTION THERAPIES: SPLANCHNIC NERVE BLOCKADE

Because an increase in SBV was identified as a major contributor to increased cardiac fillings pressures with a minimal increase in CO, splanchnic nerve blockade (SNB) was introduced.[32] This concept was first identified in the 1930s for the treatment of uncontrolled hypertension and is currently used for several indications including uncontrolled abdominal pain due to carcinoma or chronic pancreatitis.[7,33,34] Evidence indicates that long-term SNB via botulinum toxin is safe and effective in patients with refractory hypertension.[34]

Initially, SNB was attained via open surgical splanchnicectomy and later through lesser invasive thoracoscopic splanchnicectomies. In recent times, percutaneous interventions using chemical or radiofrequency ablation are in use. Reported side effects include physiological and procedural complications. A recent systematic review of 1511 published cases shows that side effects of permanent SNM resolved 48 hours after the procedure. In addition, most of the complications were reported in patients undergoing bilateral blockade.[34] Of these, the most common side effects were gastrointestinal symptoms (7.7%) followed by orthostatic hypotension (6.4%). In this case, transient orthostatic hypotension may be prevented by intense preprocedural hydration.[35] However, despite these advances, the long-term effects of SNB in patients with HF are not known (**Fig. 2**).

SHORT-TERM SPLANCHNIC NERVE BLOCKADE

The safety and efficacy of SNB have been investigated in several studies. Two small proof-of-concept studies explored the changes in SBV after SNB in patients with acute decompensated HFrEF (Splanchnic HF-1; n = 11; resting hemodynamics) and chronic HF (ambulatory HFrEF; n = 15; exercise hemodynamics).[26] SBV was simulated using heart rate, CO, PCWP, CVP, LVEF, and systolic and diastolic systemic arterial and pulmonary artery pressures. Moreover, eSBV was presented as milliliter per 70 kg body weight. Splanchnic HF-1 aimed to evaluate the effect of bilateral temporary SNB using lidocaine (duration of action <90 minutes) on CVP, PCWP, and mean PAP in patients with decompensated HFrEF. eSBV showed an average reduction of 319 ± 278 mL/70 kg while lowering right and left side cardiac filling pressures and improving CO.[26,34]

The principal aim of Splanchnic HF-2 was to measure the effect of SNM with ropivacaine (duration of action <24 hours) on exercise capacity, PCWP, and mean PAP in ambulatory patients with chronic HF.[26] This reduced resting PCWP from 27.5 ± 7.3 to 19.1 ± 8.4 mm Hg ($P < .001$), peak exercise PCWP from 34.3 ± 10.1 to 24.4 ± 10.7 mm Hg ($P < .001$) and resting systemic vascular resistance from 1676 ± 692 to 1306 ± 584 dynes/s/cm^5. In addition, cardiac index at peak exercise improved from 3.4 ± 1.2 to 3.8 ± 1.1 L/min/m^2 ($P = .011$) and peak oxygen consumption increased from 9.1 ± 2.5 to 9.8 ± 2.7 mL/kg/min ($P = .053$). Moreover, NYHA class and quality of life showed an improvement at 12 months. The eSBV is higher in decompensated patients with HFrEF than ambulatory patients with chronic HF and reduced EF ($P = .019$).[5,26] Moreover, SNB successfully reduced the eSBV in both decompensated and ambulatory HF. The majority of patients who underwent bilateral SNB reported orthostatic response to the procedure; therefore, the subsequent 10 patients underwent unilateral SNB with no reported complications[26] (Table S1).

LONG-TERM SPLANCHNIC NERVE BLOCKADE

Malek and colleagues[36] investigated the permanent surgical ablation of the splanchnic nerves in 10 patients with HFpEF using a minimally invasive thoracoscopic surgery. During a 3-month follow-up, patients showed a reduction in 20W exercise PCWP when compared with baseline −4.5 mm Hg (95% confidence interval, CI −14 to −2); $P = .0059$, which extended to peak exercise −5 mm Hg (95% CI −11–0; $P = .016$). Moreover, exercise performance borderline improved with a +1.6 mL/kg/min (95% CI, −0.3–5.7; $P = .050$) increase in peak oxygen consumption. In addition, resting CVP reduced from 10.5 (5,11) mm Hg to 6.0 (2,7) mm Hg during a 12-month follow-up.

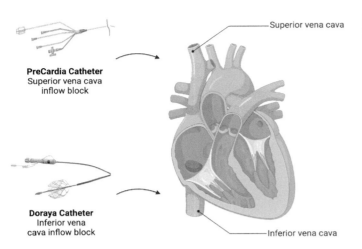

PreCardia Catheter
Superior vena cava
inflow block

Doraya Catheter
Inferior vena
cava inflow block

Superior vena cava

Inferior vena cava

Fig. 2. Timeline of splanchnic nerve blockade.

Despite the overall improved outcomes in patients with HFpEF, concerns have been raised regarding the procedural complications including surgical site infection, hematoma, and prolonged hospitalization. Therefore, a less-invasive approach, using a percutaneous nerve ablation catheter (Axon therapies) is under investigation. In a first-in-human clinical trial, Fudim and colleagues[37] used the catheter ablation system to perform endovascular catheter-based ablation of the right-sided GSN in 11 patients (3 men, 8 women) with HFpEF. There was a notable improvement in quality of life, HF severity, exercise capacity (6-minute walk test), and diastolic function. To extend these findings, a randomized, sham-controlled clinical trial (REBALANCE-HF)[38] in HFpEF is ongoing. Early results from the trial roll-in cohort (n = 18) show that all patients were treated successfully with reports of 3 nonserious moderate device/procedure-related adverse events. At a follow-up of 1 month, the mean PCWP at 20W exercise reduced from 36.4 ± 8.6 to 28.9 ± 7.8 mm Hg ($P < .01$). In addition, improvements were seen in NYHA class and KCCQ score. Therefore, the preliminary data show the safety and efficacy of catheter-based unilateral ablation of the right GSN using the catheter ablation system. These results will be confirmed in the ongoing, randomized sham-controlled portion of the trial. Another prospective open-label pilot study is underway to further investigate the safety and efficacy of long-term SNB. The Splanchnic Nerve Block for Therapy of Chronic HF (Splanchnic HF-3)[39] study will apply a long-term SNB in patients with chronic HF using botulinum toxin. The primary outcome measures are peak exercise wedge pressure, peak PAP, and absence of nerve block-related complications (see Table S1).

PRELOAD REDUCTION THERAPIES: OTHER NONPHARMACOLOGICAL INTERVENTIONS

An alternate approach for cardiac preload reduction involves unloading of the heart without changing the SBV or UBV through the translocation of blood from the pulmonary to the peripheral circulation. This may be achieved mechanically through partial or complete occlusion of the SVC or the IVC. Kaiser and colleagues[16] conducted the first-in-human study of mechanical preload reduction in 6 HFpEF patients during exercise. Balloon inflation within the IVC was performed during exercise to decrease and maintain the PAPs. Titrated partial occlusion of the IVC through balloon inflation during exercise caused a significant decline in PA pressure by 25% (from 68 ± 7 mm Hg to 51 ± 7 mm Hg) with no significant reduction in peak V_{O_2} (from 16.4 ± 5.8 mL/kg/min to 16.2 ± 4.0 mL/kg/min) or CO (14.4 ± 5.9 L/min to 12.8 ± 2.9 L/min). In addition, there was a significant reduction in respiratory rates with longer exercise times.

Further investigations have shifted focus toward novel device-based interventions for caval occlusion.[40] In a first clinical proof-of-concept study, Kapur and colleagues[41] investigated the safety and feasibility of transient SVC occlusion in patients with acutely decompensated HF and reduced ejection fraction (n = 8). SVC occlusion through a commercially available occlusion balloon for 5 minutes showed a decrease in biventricular filling pressures without any associated alterations in total CO and systemic blood pressure. A further 10-minute occlusion showed similar results in 3 of the 8 patients. In addition, patients were followed for 7-days with no reports of development of any adverse events, new neurologic symptoms, SVC injury, or thrombosis. Findings from this study have been extended to develop a catheter-mounted balloon occlusion and pump console device, known as PreCardia.

The minimally invasive PreCardia device uses a catheter-based system with an SVC balloon for intermittent occlusion of the SVC. This system has been shown to improve decongestion in acute decompensated heart failure (ADHF) by reducing cardiac filling pressures while improving renal function. The safety and efficacy of intermittent SVC occlusion using the PreCardia device in patients with ADHF is currently under investigation in the first-in-human VENUS-HF trial. Results from the early feasibility study (n = 30) show no device-related or procedure-related major adverse events in any patients during treatment of up to 24 hours. In addition, compared with baseline values, PCWP decreased by 27% (31 ± 8 vs 22 ± 9 mm Hg, $P < .001$) and right atrial pressure decreased by 34% (17 ± 4 vs 11 ± 5 mm Hg, $P < .001$). Compared with pretreatment values, the PreCardia device also increased urine output and net fluid balance by 130% and 156%, with up to 24 hours of intervention ($P < .01$).[42–44]

Majority of the patients hospitalized for acute HF present with signs and symptoms of fluid retention and are administered intravenous diuretics to ameliorate the symptoms of HF. However, up to 33% of these patients show inadequate responses to diuretics, which is a major clinical problem.[45,46] To counter this resistance to diuretics, some investigators have proposed treatment through the combination of several types of diuretics or ultrafiltration.[47,48] In a different approach, the Doraya catheter was used to treat 2 patients with ADHF showing poor diuretic response.[46] The Doraya catheter acts as a temporary intravenous flow regulator that is used percutaneously causing partial infrarenal IVC occlusion. This approach aims to trigger the unloading of the right ventricle thereby reducing cardiac preload. In addition, renal function is preserved by unloading of the renal venous system and reducing venous congestion. During this study, urine output increased from 91 mL/h to 182 mL/h. In addition, on 7 hours of follow-up, there was a reduction in CVP from 17 mm Hg to 13 mm Hg, PCWP from 29 mm Hg to 21 mm Hg, and mean PAP from 35 mm Hg to 33 mm Hg with no reports of adverse events in both patients.

To extend the findings of this investigation, a first-in-human study was conducted to ascertain the performance and safety of the Doraya catheter in patients with ADHF showing poor response to diuretic treatment and repeated volume overload.[45,49] A total of 9 patients were treated with the Doraya catheter (7 men and 2 women). There were no reports of device malfunctions or device-related adverse events or embolic events during the procedure or within 30 days of follow-up; except one case of procedure-related severe adverse event, which was resolved. Overall, the Doraya catheter decreased CVP and improved diuretic response in hospitalized patients with acute HF.

These positive results have been extended in the DORAYA-HF early feasibility study, which is expected to reach completion in 2023. Investigators aim to evaluate the safety and efficacy of the Doraya catheter in patients with ADHF with insufficient diuretic response. Primary outcomes include the occurrence of any adverse events during a period of 30 days and the urine output over 24 hours. However, it must be noted that device-based management may be used in conjunction with pharmacological therapies in patients in whom these therapies alone fail to ameliorate HF. Further investigation into the possible additive effects is needed to help guide better clinical practice. Additionally, further larger, and mid-long-term studies are required to evaluate the safety and efficacy of these devices in patient with overt systemic fluid overload and/or facts of right-sided dysfunction.

In conclusion, the SVC and IVC inflow blocks aim to improve HF outcomes without changing the SBV and UBV. This is achieved through translocation of blood out of the thoracic compartment by blocking the return of venous blood without an actual change in vascular compliance. The short-term use of these approaches has shown to improve urine output and diuretic responsiveness due to the reductions of CVP.[50] These device-based interventions allow for more effective and selective preload reduction; however, it must be noted that further investigation is needed into the longer term applications of these devices with focus on the potential complications associated with reduced blood flow to other organs, for example, the liver and kidney and device-based complications (**Fig. 3**).

In an alternate approach, investigators have explored the role of percutaneous pericardial resection for the treatment of patients with HFpEF. Initial studies in animals have shown that resection of the pericardium using a minimally invasive epicardial approach mitigates the increase in LVEDP with volume loading, thereby improving the outcomes in HFpEF patients.[51–53] A first in man pilot study[54] was conducted (n = 19) to investigate the changes in LV filling pressure (PCWP) with volume loading before and after opening the pericardium. Results showed that pericardiotomy

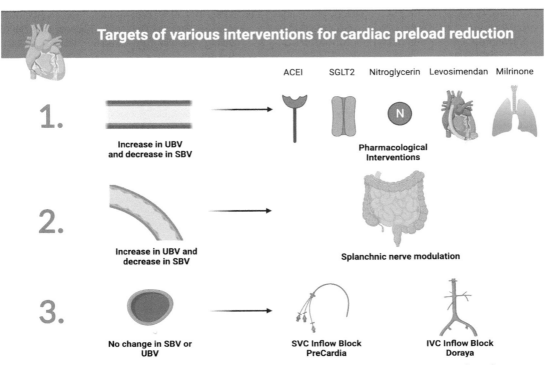

Fig. 2. Targets of device-based cardiac preload reduction therapies (PreCardia and Doraya Catheter).

without extensive pericardial resection retains the increase in LV filling pressures during volume loading in patients with risk factors for HFpEF thereby improving the outcomes. However, further investigation is warranted to evaluate the long-term safety and efficacy of this procedure in patients with HFpEF.[55]

SUMMARY

Control of cardiac preload plays a critical role in the management of acute and chronic HF. We report the emerging preload modulation therapies that include the SNB and other pharmacological and device-based therapies. Ongoing clinical trials and further investigations will extend the efficacy and safety data to help guide future clinical use and practice.

CLINICS CARE POINTS

- An increase in cardiac filling pressures can be driven by a redistribution of blood volume rather than fluid overload.
- A reduction in preload can result in an acute reduction in cardiac filling pressures.

DISCLOSURES

J. Núñez reports personal fees or advisory boards from AstraZeneca, Alleviant Medical, Boehringer Ingelheim, Bayer, Novartis, NovoNordisk, Rovi, and Vifor Pharma (outside the submitted work). M. Fudim was supported by the American Heart Association (20IPA35310955), Doris Duke, Bayer, Bodyport, and Verily. He receives consulting fees from Abbott, Ajax, Alio Health, Alleviant, Audicor, Axon-Therapies, Bayer, Bodyguide, Bodyport, Boston Scientific, Broadview, Cadence, Cardionomics, Coridea, CVRx, Daxor, Deerfield Catalyst, Edwards LifeSciences, EKO, Feldschuh Foundation, Fire1, Galvani, Gradient, Hatteras, Impulse Dynamics, Intershunt, Medtronic, Merck, NIMedical, NovoNordisk, NucleusRx, NXT Biomedical, Pharmacosmos, PreHealth, ReCor, Shifamed, Splendo, Sumacor, SyMap, Verily, Vironix, Viscardia, and Zoll.

SUPPLEMENTARY DATA

Supplementary data related to this article can be found online at https://doi.org/10.1016/j.hfc.2023.05.004.

REFERENCES

1. Rothe CF. Reflex control of veins and vascular capacitance. Physiol Rev 1983;63:1281–342.

2. Vilches, E. & Macedo Dias, A. Physiology and Path-ophysiology of Venous Flow. PanVascular Medicine, Second Edition 569–589 (2015) doi:10.1007/978-3-642-37078-6_27.

3. Burkhoff D, Tyberg Jv. Why does pulmonary venous pressure rise after onset of LV dysfunction: a theoretical analysis. Am J Physiol 1993;265.

4. Fudim M, et al. Venous Tone and Stressed Blood Volume in Heart Failure: JACC Review Topic of the Week. J Am Coll Cardiol 2022;79:1858–69.

5. Fudim M, Khan MS, Paracha AA, et al. Targeting Preload in Heart Failure: Splanchnic Nerve Blockade and Beyond. Circ Heart Fail 2022;15:211–20.

6. Wang SY, et al. Splanchnic venous pressure-volume relation during experimental acute ischemic heart failure. Differential effects of hydralazine, enalaprilat, and nitroglycerin. Circulation 1995;91:1205–12.

7. Okamoto LE, Dupont WD, Biaggioni I, et al. Effect of nitroglycerin on splanchnic and pulmonary blood volume. J Nucl Cardiol 2021. https://doi.org/10.1007/S12350-021-02811-7.

8. Sarma S, et al. Challenging the Hemodynamic Hypothesis in Heart Failure With Preserved Ejection Fraction: Is Exercise Capacity Limited by Elevated Pulmonary Capillary Wedge Pressure? Circulation 2022. https://doi.org/10.1161/CIRCULATIONAHA.122.061828.

9. Redfield MM, et al. Isosorbide Mononitrate in Heart Failure with Preserved Ejection Fraction. N Engl J Med 2015;373:2314–24.

10. Borlaug BA, et al. Latent Pulmonary Vascular Disease May Alter the Response to Therapeutic Atrial Shunt Device in Heart Failure. Circulation 2022; 145:1592–604.

11. Shah SJ, et al. Atrial shunt device for heart failure with preserved and mildly reduced ejection fraction (REDUCE LAP-HF II): a randomised, multicentre, blinded, sham-controlled trial. Lancet 2022;399:1130–40.

12. Kaye DM, Byrne M, Mariani J, et al. Identification of physiologic treatment targets with favourable haemodynamic consequences in heart failure with preserved ejection fraction. ESC Heart Fail 2020;7:3685–93.

13. Brener MI, et al. Changes in Stressed Blood Volume with Levosimendan in Pulmonary Hypertension from Heart Failure with Preserved Ejection Fraction: Insights Regarding Mechanism of Action From the HELP Trial. J Card Fail 2021;27:1023–6.

14. Omar M, et al. Effect of Empagliflozin on Blood Volume Redistribution in Patients With Chronic Heart Failure and Reduced Ejection Fraction: An Analysis from the Empire HF Randomized Clinical Trial. Circ Heart Fail 2021. https://doi.org/10.1161/CIRCHEARTFAILURE.121.009156.

15. Sorimachi H, et al. Obesity, venous capacitance, and venous compliance in heart failure with preserved ejection fraction. Eur J Heart Fail 2021;23:1648–58.

16. Kaiser DW, et al. First-in-Human Experience of Mechanical Preload Control in Patients With HFpEF During Exercise. JACC Basic Transl Sci 2021;6:189–98.

17. McCausland C, Sajjad H. Anatomy, back, splanchnic nerve. StatPearls; 2021.

18. Harper D, Chandler B. Splanchnic circulation. BJA Educ 2016;16:66–71.

19. Greenway Cv, Innes IR. Effects of splanchnic nerve stimulation on cardiac preload, afterload, and output in cats. Circ Res 1980;46:181–9.

20. Bell L, Hennecken J, Zaret BL, et al. Alpha-adrenergic regulation of splanchnic volume and cardiac output in the dog. Acta Physiol Scand 1990;138:321–9.

21. Role of splanchnic venous system in overall cardiovascular homeostasis - PubMed. Available at: https://pubmed.ncbi.nlm.nih.gov/6832386/. Accessed June, 10, 2023.

22. Role of the venous system in circulatory control - PubMed. Available at: https://pubmed.ncbi.nlm.nih.gov/345003/. Accessed June, 10, 2023.

23. Rowell LB, Detry JM, Blackmon JR, et al. Importance of the splanchnic vascular bed in human blood pressure regulation. J Appl Physiol 1972;32:213–20.

24. Fudim M, Sobotka PA, Dunlap ME. Extracardiac Abnormalities of Preload Reserve: Mechanisms Underlying Exercise Limitation in Heart Failure with Preserved Ejection Fraction, Autonomic Dysfunction, and Liver Disease. Circ Heart Fail 2021;14:2–12.

25. Fudim M, Hernandez AF, Felker GM. Role of Volume Redistribution in the Congestion of Heart Failure. J Am Heart Assoc 2017;6.

26. Fudim M, et al. Splanchnic Nerve Block Mediated Changes in Stressed Blood Volume in Heart Failure. JACC Heart Fail 2021;9:293–300.

27. Barnes RJ, Bower EA, Rink TJ. Haemodynamic responses to stimulation of the splanchnic and cardiac sympathetic nerves in the anaesthetized cat. J Physiol 1986;378:417–36.

28. Carneiro JJ, Donald DE. Change in liver blood flow and blood content in dogs during direct and reflex alteration of hepatic sympathetic nerve activity. Circ Res 1977;40:150–8.

29. Kaye DM, et al. Comprehensive Physiological Modeling Provides Novel Insights Into Heart Failure With Preserved Ejection Fraction Physiology. J Am Heart Assoc 2021;10.

30. Bapna A, Adin C, Engelman ZJ, et al. Increasing Blood Pressure by Greater Splanchnic Nerve Stimulation: a Feasibility Study. J Cardiovasc Transl Res 2020;13:509–18.

31. Fudim M, et al. Raising the pressure: Hemodynamic effects of splanchnic nerve stimulation. J Appl Physiol 2017;123:126–7.

32. Fudim M, Neuzil P, Malek F, et al. Greater Splanchnic Nerve Stimulation in Heart Failure With Preserved Ejection Fraction. J Am Coll Cardiol 2021;77:1952–3.

33. Magder S, de Varennes B. Clinical death and the measurement of stressed vascular volume. Crit Care Med 1998;26:1061–4.

34. Fudim M, et al. Splanchnic nerve modulation in heart failure: mechanistic overview, initial clinical experience, and safety considerations. Eur J Heart Fail 2021;23:1076–84.

35. Eisenberg E, Carr DB, Chalmers TC. Neurolytic celiac plexus block for treatment of cancer pain: a meta-analysis. Anesth Analg 1995;80:290–5.

36. Málek F, et al. Surgical ablation of the right greater splanchnic nerve for the treatment of heart failure with preserved ejection fraction: first-in-human clinical trial. Eur J Heart Fail 2021;23:1134–43.

37. Fudim M, et al. Transvenous Right Greater Splanchnic Nerve Ablation in Heart Failure and Preserved Ejection Fraction: First-in-Human Study. JACC Heart Fail 2022;10:744–52.

38. Fudim M, et al. Endovascular ablation of the right greater splanchnic nerve in heart failure with preserved ejection fraction: early results of the REBALANCE-HF trial roll-in cohort. Eur J Heart Fail 2022;24:1410–4.

39. Splanchnic Nerve Block for Therapy of Chronic Heart Failure (Splanchnic III) - Full Text View - ClinicalTrials.gov. Available at: https://www.clinicaltrials.gov/ct2/show/NCT04575428. Accessed June, 10, 2023.

40. Rosenblum H, et al. Conceptual Considerations for Device-Based Therapy in Acute Decompensated Heart Failure: DRI 2 P 2 S. Circ Heart Fail 2020;13.

41. Kapur NK, et al. First-in-human experience with occlusion of the superior vena cava to reduce cardiac filling pressures in congestive heart failure. Catheter Cardiovasc Interv 2019;93:1205–10.

42. SVC Occlusion in Subjects With Acute Decompensated Heart Failure - Full Text View - ClinicalTrials.gov. Available at: https://clinicaltrials.gov/ct2/show/NCT03836079. Accessed June, 10, 2023.

43. Kapur NK, et al. Intermittent Occlusion of the Superior Vena Cava Reduces Cardiac Filling Pressures in Preclinical Models of Heart Failure. J Cardiovasc Transl Res 2020;13:151–7.

44. Kapur NK, et al. Intermittent Occlusion of the Superior Vena Cava to Improve Hemodynamics in Patients With Acutely Decompensated Heart Failure: The VENUS-HF Early Feasibility Study. Circ Heart Fail 2022. https://doi.org/10.1161/CIRCHEARTFAILURE.121.008934.

45. Zymliński R, et al. Novel IVC Doraya Catheter Provides Congestion Relief in Patients With Acute Heart Failure. Basic to Translational Science 2022;7:326–7.

46. Dierckx R, et al. Treatment of Diuretic Resistance with a Novel Percutaneous Blood Flow Regulator: Concept and Initial Experience. J Card Fail 2019;25:932–4.

47. Mullens W, et al. The use of diuretics in heart failure with congestion — a position statement from the Heart Failure Association of the European Society of Cardiology. Eur J Heart Fail 2019;21:137–55.

48. Verbrugge FH, Mullens W, Tang WHW. Management of Cardio-Renal Syndrome and Diuretic Resistance. Curr Treat Options Cardiovasc Med 2016;18:1–15.

49. First In Human Study of the Doraya Catheter for the Treatment of AHF Patients - Full Text View - ClinicalTrials.gov. Available at: https://clinicaltrials.gov/ct2/show/NCT03234647. Accessed June, 10, 2023.

50. Dupont M, Mullens W, Tang WHW. Impact of systemic venous congestion in heart failure. Curr Heart Fail Rep 2011;8:233–41.

51. Percutaneous Pericardial Resection: A Novel Potential Treatment for Heart Failure with Preserved Ejection Fraction - American College of Cardiology. Available at: https://www.acc.org/latest-in-cardiology/articles/2017/09/14/12/27/percutaneous-pericardial-resection. Accessed June, 10, 2023.

52. Killu AM, et al. Beating Heart Validation of Safety and Efficacy of a Percutaneous Pericardiotomy Tool. J Cardiovasc Electrophysiol 2017;28:357–61.

53. Borlaug BA, et al. Percutaneous Pericardial Resection: A Novel Potential Treatment for Heart Failure with Preserved Ejection Fraction. Circ Heart Fail 2017;10.

54. Pericardial Resection to Treat Heart Failure - Full Text View - ClinicalTrials.gov. Available at: https://clinicaltrials.gov/ct2/show/NCT03073668. Accessed June, 10, 2023.

55. Borlaug BA, et al. Pericardiotomy Enhances Left Ventricular Diastolic Reserve with Volume Loading in Humans: Implications for the Surgical Management of Heart Failure with Preserved Ejection Fraction. Circulation 2018;138:2295.

Left Ventricular Assist Device and the Current State of the Art: HeartMate 3 at 5 Years

Omar Jawaid, MD[a], Christopher Salerno, MD[b], Ashwin Ravichandran, MD[a],*

KEYWORDS

- Heart failure • Durable mechanical support • End-stage cardiomyopathy • Outcomes

KEY POINTS

- Advanced heart failure patients have unique needs currently unmet by medical therapy alone.
- Left ventricular assist devices and heart transplantation are two strategies to help offset high mortality and morbidity in this patient population.
- Device experience and engineering have advanced tremendously in the past 20 years, resulting in fewer complications and better short- and long-term survival in these patients.

INTRODUCTION

Congestive heart failure (HF) remains the most common reason for hospitalization in the United States, with an estimated prevalence of 5.7 million people living with some sort of HF.[1] The treatment of HF with reduced ejection fraction has seen major advances in guideline medical therapy, device therapy, and improved care delivery systems. Despite these advances, however, between 5% and 10% of these patients can be categorized as having advanced HF, characterized by refractory congestive symptoms, inability to tolerate guideline therapy, hypotension, or inotrope dependence, with the largest risk factor being years since diagnosis. Advanced HF carries a dismal prognosis, with up to 50% of patients being deceased at 1 year and up to 80% at 2 years.[2] Before the advent of left ventricular assist devices (LVADs), the only treatment options for these patients were heart transplantation or palliative care. In the past 2 decades, major advances have been made with durable mechanical support systems, resulting in an additional treatment option for patients ineligible for heart transplantation.

The authors aim to describe the current state of LVAD therapy in 2023.

Indications for Implantation

The first successful LVAD was implanted in 1966 at the Methodist Hospital in Houston for a 37-year-old patient as a bridge to transplant (BTT) for 10 days. Since this landmark event, over 27,000 devices have been implanted for end-stage HF as defined by the New York Heart Association (NYHA) classification system. LVADs are implanted as a BTT for patients either too sick or otherwise ineligible for primary transplant, or as destination therapy (DT), in which transplantation is not an option.[3,4] The current state-of-the-art device, the HeartMate 3 (Abbott Corporation, North Chicago, IL), is a magnetically levitated centrifugal-flow device and currently constitutes the majority of devices implanted contemporaneously in the United States. Prior devices, including the HeartMate-XVE (Thoratec Corp, Pleasanton, CA), Novacor N100 (Baxter Healthcare Corporation, Novacor Division, Oakland, CA), HeartMate 2 (Thoratec Corp, Pleasanton, CA), and HeartWare (HVAD, Medtronic Inc, Minnesota, MN), are no

a St. Vincents' Ascension, 8333 Naab Road, Indianapolis, IN 46260, USA; b University of Chicago Medical Center, 5841 South Maryland Avenue, Chicago, IL 60637, USA
* Corresponding author.
E-mail address: ashwin.ravichandran@ascension.org

Heart Failure Clin 20 (2024) 83–89
https://doi.org/10.1016/j.hfc.2023.05.005
1551-7136/24/© 2023 Elsevier Inc. All rights reserved.

heartfailure.theclinics.com

longer implanted de novo and thus are considered legacy devices as of 2023 in the United States.

LVAD therapy is considered once patients demonstrate signs and symptoms of end-stage HF, indicated by an ejection fraction less than 25%, worsening symptoms despite escalating therapy, multiple HF hospitalizations, inability to tolerate guideline therapy, hypotension, end-organ dysfunction, including kidney and liver injury, cachexia, and/or a need for inotropic therapy to maintain perfusion, thereby improving HF symptoms. This patient population derives the most benefit from LVAD implantation at an acceptable risk: benefit ratio with regard to adverse events.[5,6]

As a BTT, LVADs are used to stabilize end-organ function and maintain viability as a transplant candidate, whereas DT LVAD patients receive the device as the definitive treatment of their HF. Originally designed as BTT therapy, the 2018 United Network for Organ Sharing (UNOS) organ reallocation revision for heart transplantation impacted patient selection for LVAD implantation. Before 2018, up to 47% of patients receiving an LVAD were implanted as a BTT. Now, 81% of LVAD implants are placed as a DT indication.[4] This is in part due to the new allocation system de-prioritizing stable LVAD patients in favor of sicker patients who need an organ more urgently. These patients are now listed as status 4, representing otherwise stable LVAD recipients. In contrast, most organs are now allocated to those listed status 1, 2, or 3, representing patients with the most hemodynamic compromise requiring extracorporeal membrane oxygenation, temporary mechanical support, or high-dose inotropes with invasive hemodynamic monitoring.[4] As the rate of DT implantation has increased, so too has the average age of implanted patients, rising to an average age of 56.7 years in 2021 versus 53 years in 2008.

Patient selection remains a key aspect of LVAD implantation. Ideally, patients are referred to advanced HF centers once it becomes evident that medical therapy is no longer sufficient. Using mnemonics such as "I NEED HELP" (**Table 1**) can aid decision-making in referring these patients to centers specializing in LVAD and heart transplantation. A synthesis of clinical, biochemical, and hemodynamic data is needed before the decision is made to proceed with durable mechanical support. The 2006 International Society for Heart/Lung Transplant (ISHLT) guidelines emphasize the need for cardiopulmonary exercise (CPEX) testing to help guide decision-making, with a peak VO2 max of less than 14 mL/kg/min, or less than 12 mL/kg/min on beta blocker therapy, strongly suggesting the need for heart transplantation and has since been extrapolated to LVAD therapy.[6–9] In addition, patients being considered for LVAD therapy should

Table 1 Markers of advanced heart failure	
I	*Inotropes*
N	*NYHA IV/high n-terminal pro-brain natriuretic peptide (NT-proBNP)*
E	*End-organ dysfunction*
E	*Ejection fraction <25%*
D	*Defibrillator shocks*
H	More than two *hospitalizations* in 6 months
E	*Edema/escalating diuretics for refractory symptoms*
L	*Low blood pressure*
P	*Prognostic medications, inability to tolerate or removal of guideline therapy*

also not have significant competing causes for morbidity and mortality such as metastatic cancer, end-stage renal disease, cirrhosis, or incurable infectious disease.[6,8] Patients who meet the definition for frailty may not benefit from LVAD implantation due to poor functional status from comorbid conditions such as diabetes, peripheral vascular disease, anemia as well as through an internally validated questionnaire. In this population, patients with the highest frailty indices had a 1-year mortality of close to 40% post-VAD.[10] Finally, consideration of psychosocial situation, history of current substance abuse, and caregiver support should be undertaken before committing to LVAD implant due to the significant caregiver and patient burden needed to maintain the device as well as frequent laboratory and clinic visits.[6,8] Thus, a careful selection must be undertaken to identify patients most likely to benefit while providing equitable treatment to populations from varied social and economic backgrounds.

Left Ventricular Assist Device Benefits

In 2001, the HeartMate-Vented Electric (VE) was demonstrated to be superior as compared with contemporary medical therapy in the landmark REMATCH trial with 52% of patients surviving at 1-year versus just 25% of patients on medical therapy alone.[11] Since then, subsequent device trials have demonstrated continued improved survival in NYHA class IV patients as well as quality of life improvements. The HeartMate 3 device demonstrated superiority to the HeartMate 2 device at 2 years in the Momentum-3 trial driven by lower rates of device failure in the form of pump thrombosis (1.4% vs 13.9%) as well as device complications, including gastrointestinal bleeding (43.7% vs 55%), stroke (9.9% vs 19.4%), and pump exchanges (2.3% vs 11.3%). In the modern era, early survival now rivals transplant, with up to 85% of patients being alive after 2 years.[12] Recently, 5-year survival data for the HeartMate 3 was published and demonstrated superiority over HeartMate 2 patients as observed in an extension study of the Momentum-3 trial. At 5 years, 54% of HeartMate 3 patients were still alive, compared with 30% of HeartMate 2 patients.[13] Moreover, the outside of randomized clinical trials, continued access protocol (CAP), and registry level data demonstrate similar results at 2 years in the HeartMate 3 implant population. Similar to Momentum-3, under a CAP, nearly 1700 NYHA IV patients were implanted with a HeartMate 3 as either BTT or DT. These patients demonstrated similar rates of survival at 2 years, with 81.2% survival. Rates of bleeding, stroke, and pump thrombosis were also similar to clinical trial patients. Likewise, the ELEVATE registry, which studied predominantly a European population of 540 advanced HF patients, demonstrated 74.5% survival at 2 years with similar rates of reported bleeding and stroke at 33.3% and 10.7%, respectively.[14,15] Both CAP enrollment and ELEVATE registry demonstrate the generalizability of this device to the large advanced HF population and not carefully selected clinical trial participants.

Ambulatory advanced HF patients, defined as those not requiring inotropic therapy, and otherwise qualified for device therapy, were studied in the ROADMAP study. Advanced NYHA IIIb or IV patients were observed with respect to early HeartMate 2 implantation versus medical therapy. Within 1 year, 80% of HeartMate 2 patients were alive versus 63% of medical therapy patients. Moreover, implanted patients demonstrated improved quality of life as measured by the EuroQOL 5-dimensional questionnaire (EQ-5D) VAS questionnaire, demonstrating an average improvement of 29 points as compared with 10 points in the medical therapy arm.[5]

Using data from the HeartMate 2 trials, both renal and hepatic indices improved post-LVAD implant and was sustained for 6 months, often normalizing as adequate circulation is restored despite concerns over nonphysiologic nonpulsatile blood flow adversely impacting end-organ function. This is likely in part due to improved cardiac output as well as effective decongestion.[16,17] This effect persists to 3 years post-implant, with glomerular filtration rate (GFR) being approximately 2% above pre-implant levels in this population and with hepatic indices remaining in the normal range at 3 years post-therapy.[17]

In addition to mortality benefits and biochemical indices improvements, LVAD implantation results in significant quality of life benefits. In a study using CPEX testing, patients were able to achieve a VO2 max of 23 mL/kg/min 12 weeks after implantation, improved from an average of 10 mL/kg/min before implantation. This finding was like those post-heart transplantation at 1 year.[18] Assessments of quality of life by various surveys also demonstrate significant benefit after LVAD implantation. At 3 and 6 months post-implant, respondents to the Kansas City Cardiomyopathy questionnaire demonstrated a marked improvement of 19 points. Likewise, respondents to the Minnesota Living with Heart Failure Questionnaire demonstrated similar improvements after HM2 implantation, with scores dropping more than 50% as compared with pre-implant values. Moreover, this benefit was seen regardless of LVAD implant indication (BTT or DT). Underscoring the need for proper patient selection, elderly patients did not demonstrate a significant improvement in quality of life until much later, at 12 months post-implant.[19] The type of LVAD did not seemingly impact quality of life measurements as both HM2 and HM3 devices resulted in similar improvements,[12] underscoring that relief of symptoms often drives benefit. However, freedom from complications, including gastrointestinal bleeding, stroke, and device exchanges were markedly lower in patients implanted with the HeartMate 3 device.[12]

Thrombosis and Stroke

Although LVAD therapy remains a life-saving intervention for those with end-stage HF, it comes with risks and known complications including gastrointestinal bleeding, ischemic and hemorrhagic strokes, driveline infections, and right HF. Devices have become more hemocompatible with each iteration, though the need for systemic anticoagulation remains.

Pump thrombosis and stroke rates in the HeartMate 3 pump are dramatically reduced due to the improved engineering design of the newer generation device using magnetically levitated motors, wider inflow cannula gaps, and intrinsic pulsatile function. This results in improved hemocompatibility as fewer moving parts are exposed to blood as well reduced shear stress and heat generation, reducing the risk of pump thrombosis, device exchange, and strokes. Approximately 10% of HeartMate 2 devices were exchanged at 2 years, as compared with 2% for HeartMate 3.[12] This benefit was maintained out to 5 years, with pump thrombosis rates of 0.01 events per patient-year in the HeartMate 3 group as compared with 0.108 events per patient-year in patients implanted with the HeartMate 2,[13] allowing for investigation into liberalization of anticoagulation and antiplatelet regimens to provide more personalized care for the LVAD patient.

However, despite improved hemocompatibility with fewer bleeding and thromboembolic complications, stroke still remains a major contributor of morbidity and mortality in the LVAD population. In the current generation of devices, the HeartMate 3 demonstrated superiority over prior devices in the rate of strokes, with approximately one-third fewer strokes as compared with HeartMate 2 devices.[12] Stroke remains one of the major causes of morbidity and mortality, with up to 24% of patients experiencing a stroke preceding death.[20] Risk factors include inability to tolerate anticoagulation, labile international normalized ratio (INR), and hypertension.[20,21] Up to 63% of strokes were ischemic or thromboembolic in nature with the remainder being hemorrhagic.[21] Unlike gastrointestinal (GI) bleeding, the management of strokes in this population is still developing. Tissue plasminogen activator is generally considered contraindicated due to concerns over hemorrhagic conversion, and thrombectomy is poorly studied in this patient population.[22,23]

Bleeding and Infection

LVADs predispose patients to both thrombosis and bleeding complications. Owing to hemocompatibility concerns, therapeutic anticoagulation is pursued whenever feasible. In addition, LVADs remove pulsatile flow, which is theorized to predispose to the formation of arteriovenous malformations. Thus, patients are rehospitalized often for gastrointestinal bleeding, affecting 18% to 40% of patients implanted. The cause of GI bleeding is multifactorial, including loss of pulsatile blood flow, increased endothelial fragility, need for systemic anticoagulation, abnormal von Willebrand factor multimers, and platelet dysfunction.[24] GI bleeding remains a leading cause of early and late rehospitalization in these patients, accounting for up to 16% of the primary reason why patients are readmitted within 30 days.[25] The HeartMate 3 demonstrated superiority over the HeartMate 2 with respect to GI bleeding at 2 years post-implant, though event rates remained elevated at 0.31 events per patient-year.[12] At the 5-year mark, this reduction in GI bleeding remained durable, with the HeartMate 3 demonstrating a near 60% reduction in GI bleeding events, at 0.252 events per patient-year versus 0.423 events per patient-year in the HeartMate 2.[13] The ARIES trial, which recently completed enrollment, will also help answer the question regarding the need for aspirin therapy in the current HeartMate 3 era,[26]

thereby lowering overall propensity for bleeding in these patients.

Driveline infections remain distressingly common. Studies on prevalence of infection estimate 14% to 48% patients will have a driveline infection during the lifespan of their device. As drivelines exit the body, they create a nidus for infection that often becomes colonized with biofilm. Lacking a vascular supply, control of the infection can be difficult, often resulting in long-term intravenous or suppressive antibiotics. Unfortunately, driveline infections can progress to device infections, with corresponding increase in mortality and morbidity, and the only cure is often device exchange.[27,28] Overall rates of infection do not differ between the Heartmate 2 and Heartmate 3, with near identical 5-year infection rates at 0.551 and 0.515 events per patient-year, respectively[13] (**Table 2**).

Future of Left Ventricular Assist Device Therapy

Although LVADs are life-saving devices, implantation has been on the decline over the past 3 years. Because the UNOS 2018 organ reallocation changes, BTT implants have declined drastically, from 48.9% in 2018 to 6.6% in 2021. Accordingly, the total number of devices declined from an all-time high of 3219 in 2018 to 2464 in 2022.[4] No doubt, the ongoing COVID-19 pandemic has played a role, though heart transplantation has remained steady despite the pandemic.[29] Of note, African American and female patients are implanted at lower frequencies than their Caucasian counterparts.[30] Women represent only 20% of LVAD recipients despite similar representations across the spectrum of HF.[2] Likewise, black patients were

Table 2 HeartMate 2 versus HeartMate 3 at 5 years		
	HeartMate 2	**HeartMate 3**
Survival (%)	43.70%	*58.40%*
Pump thrombosis (event/patient-years)	0.108	*0.01*
Stroke (event/patient-years)	0.136	*0.05*
Bleeding (event/patient-years)	0.765	*0.43*
Infection (event/patient-years)	0.551	0.5145
$P<.05$		

Advanced Heart Failure
- Incidence of 2–5% of heart failure population
- Few medical therapies to reduce mortality and morbidity.
- LVAD or Heart Transplantation however availability of hearts outweigh need.

Current state of the art in LVAD Technology
- HeartMate 3 (HM3) as dominant implant today.
- Dramatic improvement past 20 y
  - Improved short- and long-term mortality across device iterations.
  - HM3 at 5-y significant mortality and morbidity benefit vs HM2.

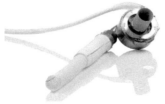

Device complication profile continues to improve
- HeartMate3 vs HeartMate2
  - Fewer strokes due to improved hemocompatibility
  - Less incident GI bleeding
  - Improved pump thrombosis rates
  - Improved ability to tailor anticoagulation regimens to balance bleeding/thrombosis risk.

Future of LVAD technology
- Several devices in clinical and pre-clinical trials
- Continued hemocompatibility advancements
- Improve hemodynamic profile
- Improve access to women and minority patients

Fig. 1. Overview of the current landscape of the HeartMate 3 LVAD. (Reproduced with permission from Impulse Dynamics.)

6% less likely to receive an LVAD, though this trend has reversed in later years.[30,31] Given this need for advanced therapies in historically underrepresented populations, there are great opportunities for increased access even as overall implant volumes decrease. Timely referral for patients remains the most important aspect in determining candidacy and access to these life-saving devices.

The past 10 years have seen significant changes in the LVAD space. The advent of magnetically levitated rotors has drastically improved hemocompatibility as compared with prior axial rotor devices as reflected by reduced stroke, pump thrombosis, and GI bleeding rates, though significant residual risk remains. In addition, the LVAD market has seen drastic changes with the HVAD device being recalled in 2021 by the Food and Drug Administration (FDA) due to controller, battery, and unpredictable pump stoppages, with the manufacturer voluntarily removing the device from the market in 2021. As a result, the HeartMate 3 is the only device being implanted actively in the United States.[4,32]

Looking toward the future, the Evaheart (EVA2) device is currently in randomized controlled trials against the HeartMate 3.[33] The study investigators aim to randomize almost 400 patients and should be completed around 2024, though the COVID-19 pandemic likely has delayed this. The EVA2 device is a smaller pump that boasts a seamless inflow cannula that implants flush with the surface of the left ventricle, reportedly improving the hemocompatibility, as reducing right ventricular failure post-implant by causing less suction of the septum by LVAD inflow cannula.[34] At this time, no other devices are being implanted in patients, though several devices are currently in preclinical testing

phases, such as the CorWave, CH-ventricular assist device (CH-VAD), and the total artificial heart, BiVaCor.[35–37] This is a rapidly evolving space, and no doubt innovation in the future will reduce complications and improve outcomes as each successive generation has done so (**Fig. 1**).

The last 20 years have been a whirlwind of progress in the durable mechanical support realm and this hints toward the progress anticipated in the next 20 years. Although complication rates have decreased dramatically, they often remain unacceptably high for many patients, limiting overall uptake of these devices. Innovations to eliminate the external driveline, to improve the hemocompatibility further, as well as potentially durable right-sided support are outstanding issues that will need to be addressed in future iterations of these devices. Although 2-year survival rivals that of transplant, long-term survival remains inferior to transplant. As the availability of organs limits transplant volumes, the nature of LVADs being readily available offers a tantalizing solution to meet the needs of the advanced HF population.

CLINICS CARE POINTS

- Timely referral of advanced heart failure patients is a key in providing the best outcomes; patients unable to tolerate medical therapy, hypotension, or multiple admissions should be referred to an advanced heart failure center.
- Successive device iterations have reduced complication rates and improved survival rates over the past 2 decades; the current

HeartMate 3 offers more than 50% survival at 5 years with reduced rates of bleeding, stroke, and pump thrombosis.

- Advanced heart failure centers are uniquely positioned to care for these complex patients.

DISCLOSURE

O. Jawaid has no relevant disclosures. A. Ravichandran has no relevant disclosures. C. Salerno has no relevant disclosures.

REFERENCES

1. Akintoye E, Briasoulis A, Egbe A, et al. National trends in admission and in-hospital mortality of patients with heart failure in the United States (2001-2014). J Am Heart Assoc 2017;6(12):e006955.
2. Subramaniam AV, Weston SA, Killian JM, et al. Development of advanced heart failure: a population-based study. Circ Heart Fail 2022;15(5): e009218.
3. Teuteberg JJ, Cleveland JC Jr, Cowger J, et al. The society of thoracic surgeons intermacs 2019 annual report: the changing landscape of devices and indications. Ann Thorac Surg 2020;109(3):649–60.
4. Yuzefpolskaya M, Schroeder SE, Houston BA, et al. The society of thoracic surgeons Intermacs 2022 annual report: focus on the 2018 heart transplant allocation system. Ann Thorac Surg 2023;115(2): 311–27.
5. Starling RC, Estep JD, Horstmanshof DA, et al, ROADMAP Study Investigators. Risk assessment and comparative effectiveness of left ventricular assist device and medical management in ambulatory heart failure patients: the ROADMAP study 2-year results. JACC Heart Fail 2017;5(7):518–27.
6. Guglin M, Zucker MJ, Borlaug BA, et al. ACC heart failure and transplant member section and leadership council. evaluation for heart transplantation and LVAD implantation: JACC council perspectives. J Am Coll Cardiol 2020;75(12):1471–87.
7. Mehra MR, Kobashigawa J, Starling R, et al. Listing criteria for heart transplantation: International Society for Heart and Lung Transplantation guidelines for the care of cardiac transplant candidates–2006. J Heart Lung Transplant 2006;25(9):1024–42.
8. Kirklin JK, Pagani FD, Goldstein DJ, et al. American association for thoracic surgery/international society for heart and lung transplantation guidelines on selected topics in mechanical circulatory support. J Thorac Cardiovasc Surg 2020;159(3):865–96.
9. Caraballo C, DeFilippis EM, Nakagawa S, et al. Clinical outcomes after left ventricular assist device implantation in older adults: an INTERMACS analysis. JACC Heart Fail 2019;7(12):1069–78.
10. Dunlay SM, Park SJ, Joyce LD, et al. Frailty and outcomes after implantation of left ventricular assist device as destination therapy. J Heart Lung Transplant 2014;33(4):359–65.
11. Rose EA, Gelijns AC, Moskowitz AJ, et al. Randomized evaluation of mechanical assistance for the treatment of congestive heart failure (REMATCH) study group. Long-term use of a left ventricular assist device for end-stage heart failure. N Engl J Med 2001;345(20):1435–43.
12. Mehra MR, Uriel N, Naka Y, et al. MOMENTUM 3 Investigators. A Fully Magnetically Levitated Left Ventricular Assist Device - Final Report. N Engl J Med 2019;380(17):1618–27.
13. Mehra MR, Goldstein DJ, Cleveland JC, et al. Five-year outcomes in patients with fully magnetically levitated vs axial-flow left ventricular assist devices in the MOMENTUM 3 randomized trial. JAMA 2022;328(12):1233–42.
14. Mehra MR, Cleveland JC Jr, Uriel N, et al. MOMENTUM 3 Investigators. Primary results of long-term outcomes in the MOMENTUM 3 pivotal trial and continued access protocol study phase: a study of 2200 HeartMate 3 left ventricular assist device implants. Eur J Heart Fail 2021;23(8):1392–400.
15. Zimpfer D, Gustafsson F, Potapov E, et al. Two-year outcome after implantation of a full magnetically levitated left ventricular assist device: results from the ELEVATE Registry. Eur Heart J 2020;41(39):3801–9.
16. Yoshioka D, Takayama H, Colombo PC, et al. Changes in End-Organ Function in Patients With Prolonged Continuous-Flow Left Ventricular Assist Device Support. Ann Thorac Surg 2017 Mar; 103(3):717–24.
17. Russell SD, Rogers JG, Milano CA, et al. HeartMate II Clinical Investigators. Renal and hepatic function improve in advanced heart failure patients during continuous-flow support with the HeartMate II left ventricular assist device. Circulation 2009;120(23): 2352–7.
18. de Jonge N, Kirkels H, Lahpor JR, et al. Exercise performance in patients with end-stage heart failure after implantation of a left ventricular assist device and after heart transplantation: an outlook for permanent assisting? J Am Coll Cardiol 2001;37(7): 1794–9.
19. Maciver J, Rao V, Ross HJ. Quality of life for patients supported on a left ventricular assist device. Expert Rev Med Devices 2011;8(3):325–37.
20. Dunlay SM, Strand JJ, Wordingham SE, et al. Dying with a left ventricular assist device as destination therapy. Circ Heart Fail 2016;9(10):e003096.
21. Inamullah O, Chiang YP, Bishawi M, et al. Characteristics of strokes associated with centrifugal flow left ventricular assist devices. Sci Rep 2021;11(1):1645.

22. Rettenmaier LA, Garg A, Limaye K, et al. Management of ischemic stroke following left ventricular assist device. J Stroke Cerebrovasc Dis 2020; 29(12):105384.

23. Rogers JG, Pagani FD, Tatooles AJ, et al. Intrapericardial left ventricular assist device for advanced heart failure. N Engl J Med 2017;376(5):451–60.

24. Vedachalam S, Balasubramanian G, Haas GJ, et al. Treatment of gastrointestinal bleeding in left ventricular assist devices: a comprehensive review. World J Gastroenterol 2020;26(20):2550–8.

25. Agrawal S, Garg L, Shah M, et al. Thirty-day readmissions after left ventricular assist device implantation in the United States: insights from the nationwide readmissions database. Circ Heart Fail 2018;11(3):e004628.

26. Mehra MR, Crandall DL, Gustafsson F, et al. Aspirin and left ventricular assist devices: rationale and design for the international randomized, placebo-controlled, non-inferiority ARIES HM3 trial. Eur J Heart Fail 2021;23(7):1226–37.

27. Leuck AM. Left ventricular assist device driveline infections: recent advances and future goals. J Thorac Dis 2015;7(12):2151–7.

28. O'Horo JC, Abu Saleh OM, Stulak JM, et al. Left ventricular assist device infections: a systematic review. ASAIO J 2018;64(3):287–94.

29. Available at: https://unos.org/news/in-focus/heart-transplant-all-time-record-2021/. Accessed March 13, 2023.

30. Cascino TM, Somanchi S, Colvin M, et al. Racial and sex inequities in the use of and outcomes after left ventricular assist device implantation among medicare beneficiaries. JAMA Netw Open 2022;5(7): e2223080.

31. Breathett K, Allen LA, Helmkamp L, et al. Temporal trends in contemporary use of ventricular assist devices by race and ethnicity. Circ Heart Fail 2018; 11(8):e005008.

32. Available at: https://www.fda.gov/medical-devices/cardiovascular-devices/recalls-related-hvad-system#:~: text=FDA%20Activities%20Related%20to%20the%20 HVAD%20System,-Date&text=The%20FDA%20 issued%20a%20recall,internal%20component%20 as%20Class%201. Accessed March 13, 2023.

33. Available at: https://clinicaltrials.gov/ct2/show/NCT01187368. Accessed March 13, 2023.

34. Available at: https://www.evaheart-usa.com/. Accessed March 13, 2023.

35. Botterbusch C, Barabino N, Cornat F, et al. Progress in the development of the pulsatile CorWave LVAD. J Heart Lung Transplant 2021;40(4, Supplement): S104.

36. Available at: https://us.chbiomedical.com/product/CH_VAD.aspx. Accessed March 12, 2023.

37. Available at: https://bivacor.com/. Accessed March 12, 2023.

Targeted Therapies for Microvascular Disease

Adam Bland, MBBS[a,b], Eunice Chuah, MBBS[a,b], William Meere, MBBS[a,b],
Thomas J. Ford, MBChB (Hons), PhD[a,b,c,]*

KEYWORDS

• CMD • INOCA • Angina • Ischemia • Management

KEY POINTS

- Coronary microvascular dysfunction (CMD) is a common cause of ischemia in patients without obstructive coronary artery disease (INOCA). CMD typically results from impaired vasodilation and/or excessive vasoconstriction.
- Invasive assessment of the coronary microcirculation can stratify anti-ischemic therapy to improved patient outcomes. Beta-blockers are the cornerstone of therapy for angina with CMD.
- Management of CMD includes a combination of pharmacological therapy and cardiovascular risk factor modification including lifestyle interventions. Pharmacological treatment may be divided into antiatherosclerotic therapy and antianginal therapy.
- Further randomized clinical trials are required to determine effects of current management strategies, as well as proposed novel therapies.

INTRODUCTION

Coronary artery disease (CAD) is a leading cause of morbidity and mortality affecting 126 million worldwide individuals (approaching 2% of the earth's population).[1] Obstructive epicardial CAD has been the focus of most research in the era of percutaneous coronary intervention (PCI). Patients with ischemia but no obstructive coronary artery disease (INOCA) have largely been overlooked until recently in part related to challenges in diagnosis, poorly understood pathophysiology, and lack of standardised diagnostic criteria.[2] Coronary microvascular dysfunction (CMD) is one endotype of INOCA along with vasospastic angina, mixed INOCA, and noncardiac chest pain.[3] Chest pain with no obstructive CAD previously was under the umbrella term of cardiac syndrome X (CSX); however, INOCA is now a preferred umbrella term replacing the ambiguous term CSX in recognition of better

understanding of the endotypes that may coexist to drive myocardial ischemia.[4,5]

Approximately 50% of diagnostic coronary angiograms for patients at high risk of CAD demonstrate unobstructed coronary arteries. Many of these patients have abnormal stress testing, unstable angina, and non-ST-elevation myocardial infarction.[6,7] Up to two-thirds of INOCA patients undergoing functional coronary angiography are subsequently demonstrated to have CMD, diagnosed by demonstrating reduced coronary flow reserve (CFR), and/or elevated microvascular resistance.[8] Noninvasive testing of these patients often shows reduced myocardial perfusion reserve on cardiac MRI or PET.[8–10] INOCA is a particularly relevant diagnosis in women presenting with angina in whom unobstructed coronary arteries is a more common finding than in their male counterparts.[11] The COVADIS working group has helped with some unifying definitions including microvascular

This article originally appeared in *Interventional Cardiology Clinics*, Volume 12, Issue 1, January 2023.
[a] Department of Cardiology, Gosford Hospital - Central Coast LHD, 75 Holden Street, Gosford, New South Wales 2250, Australia; [b] The University of Newcastle, University Dr, Callaghan, New South Wales 2308, Australia; [c] University of Glasgow, ICAMS, G12 8QQ Glasgow, UK
* Corresponding author. Department of Cardiology, Gosford Hospital - Central Coast LHD, 75 Holden Street, Gosford, New South Wales 2250, Australia.
E-mail address: Tom.ford@health.nsw.gov.au

Heart Failure Clin 20 (2024) 91–99
https://doi.org/10.1016/j.hfc.2023.06.003
1551-7136/24/

angina (MVA) which refers to angina patients without flow-limiting CAD but in whom invasive or noninvasive tests show evidence of CMD[12,13] (**Fig. 1**).

Despite the absence of epicardial obstruction, CMD remains associated with higher major adverse cardiovascular events (MACE) including cardiovascular mortality, as well as higher repeat angiography, higher levels of depression and lower quality of life.[2,9,12,14–16] Patients with CMD, however, remain largely undertreated due to difficulties over recent decades in establishing a widely accepted diagnostic criteria, and subsequently large trials and guidelines addressing CMD management are lacking.[9,17,18] This review aims to discuss the evolving management of CMD including the role of targeted therapies.

TREATMENT TARGETS FOR MICROVASCULAR DYSFUNCTION

Coronary blood flow incorporates 3 distinct compartments. Larger epicardial arteries appreciable on diagnostic coronary angiogram range from approximately 500 μm up to 5 mm or greater.[18,19] The microcirculation consists of intermediate pre-arterioles (~100–500 μm diameter), and smaller intramural arterioles (<100 μm in diameter).[18,19] The coronary microcirculation alters blood flow to meet cardiac myocyte metabolic demand, with increased demand and flow causing vasodilation, and decreased demand and flow causing vasoconstriction. Proximal arteriolar stretch receptors or distal arteriolar local metabolites dictate these alterations in arteriolar size.[18]

CMD results from an inability of the microvasculature to meet cardiac myocyte demand, resulting in ischemia and angina. Traditional cardiovascular risk factors remain the same for CMD including hypertension, dyslipidemia, diabetes mellitus, ageing, and smoking.[18] However, CMD also has significant predisposition for women.[3,16,20] Aggressive reversible risk factor modification, although limited in evidence, is accepted to be fundamental to CMD management.[3,18,21] CMD is also associated with increased mild epicardial atherosclerosis, which may suggest a reason for increased levels of MACE associated with this disorder but further highlights the need for risk factor optimization.[22,23] Other specific disorders predispose to microvascular dysfunction including hypertrophic cardiomyopathy and idiopathic dilated cardiomyopathy. Treatment of these unique situations is outside the scope of this review.

CMD is heterogenous in its pathophysiology, clinical presentation, and response to therapy.[3] The inability of the coronary microcirculation to meet cardiac myocyte demand in CMD can be because of excessive vasoconstriction, or inadequate vasodilation.[24] Invasive angiographic provocation testing can help direct and individualize pharmacological therapy for CMD. Endothelial dysfunction results in vasoconstriction and can be demonstrated with intracoronary acetylcholine during coronary angiography.[24] Epicardial vasoconstriction detected with acetylcholine represents vasospastic angina, which can coexist with CMD, and is best treated with calcium channel blockade.[25] If there is no epicardial vasoconstriction to acetylcholine, but symptoms or electrocardiogram signs of ischemia are reproduced (or to adenosine), this indicates endothelial-dependent CMD and again suggests likely benefit to calcium channel blockade.[24]

CFR is the ratio of coronary blood flow at maximal dilation (commonly after intracoronary adenosine) compared with blood flow at baseline, which is reduced in CMD. It suggests impaired ability of the microvasculature to dilate and accommodate increased coronary flow during demand resulting in angina.[18] This is termed endothelial-independent CMD.[24] Beta-blockers are the recommended first line for CMD, especially when impaired vasodilation is suspected.[21] Subsequently, individuals with mixed endothelial-independent CMD and either endothelial-dependent CMD or vasospastic angina require combination therapy.[17] Confirming the diagnosis

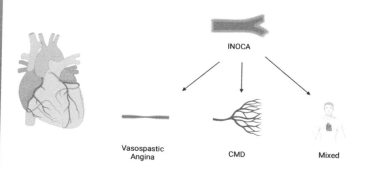

Fig. 1. INOCA endotypes.

of CMD at time of angiography and titrating therapy to the endotype of CMD has demonstrated patient benefits including improved angina and quality of life[26] (**Fig. 2**).

Given the lack of large clinical trials, the management of CMD is based on weak evidence and much of the direction for treatment has been made from trials concerning INOCA or CSX. These pathologic conditions do not exclude vasospastic angina and some noncardiac causes of chest pain, rendering them unreliable when applying to CMD.[24] Despite this, widely accepted management principles include a combination of risk factor modification, antiatherosclerotic therapy, and antiangina therapy.[17] Novel therapies are being trialled for this chronic disorder without a cure, particularly as some individuals may have limited benefit to standard care resulting in significant residual morbidity and poor quality of life.

Reversible Risk Factors

Cardiac rehabilitation and physical exercise
Although outside the scope of this review of pharmacological therapy, the role of physical activity and cardiac rehabilitation cannot be emphasized enough. Cardiac rehabilitation may help with illness understanding[27] and alleviate some of the understandable fear that comes with a diagnosis of angina. Neuromodulation in this way may improve symptoms and alleviate anxiety to reduce pain.[28] Cardiac rehabilitation has been shown to have benefit in coronary angina, and exercise has been demonstrated to improve endothelial dysfunction.[29] A small trial of 13 subjects completed a 6-week cardiovascular conditioning program and a low-fat diet, which demonstrated improved myocardial flow reserve through improving vasodilatory capacity and resting blood flow.[30] A systematic review involving 8 trials looking at exercise prescription for angina in individuals with nonobstructive CAD showed improvements in oxygen uptake, angina severity, exercise capacity and quality of life.[31] Although this is not specifically CMD and may include patients with vasospastic angina, it would suggest likely benefit in the CMD population.

Hypertension
Hypertension is associated with lower CFR and subsequent predisposition to CMD.[32] A trial with 137 subjects demonstrated treatment with

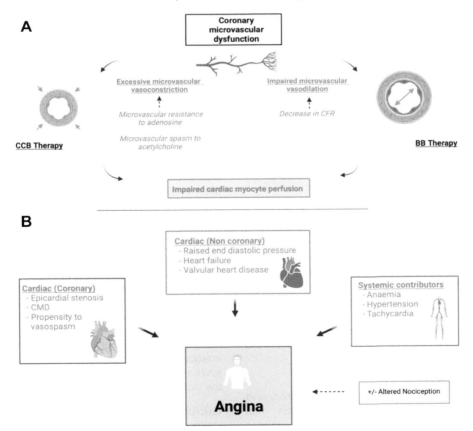

Fig. 2. CMD pathophysiology, therapy, and contributions to angina.

antihypertensive therapy down to a normal blood pressure significantly improves CFR suggesting microvascular functional improvement but this data did not capture angina change.[32] Perindopril therapy in 14 hypertensive patients for 12 months has demonstrated regression of periarteriolar fibrosis and improvement in coronary reserve.[33]

Dyslipidemia
Inverse correlations were observed between CFR and total lipid levels including low density lipoprotein (LDL) using PET scanning, suggesting LDL can contribute to CMD.[34] In another study, 25 patients with familial hypercholesterolemia were found to have significant reduction in myocardial blood flow and CFR using PET scanning.[35]

Smoking
In a study with 354 subjects, smoking has been shown to be associated with a significant reduction in transthoracic echocardiogram detected CFR, suggesting microvascular dysfunction.[36] Furthermore, another small trial with 19 subjects demonstrated and average reduced CFR of 21% using PET scan in smokers, which improved following vitamin C to suggest oxidative stress is likely involved in some element of pathogenesis of CMD.[18,37]

Diabetes mellitus
Microvascular dysfunction is a known feature of diabetes resulting in retinopathy, nephropathy, and neuropathy.[18] Type 1 and 2 diabetes mellitus have been shown to have reduced coronary vasodilator function predisposing to CMD.[38] Obesity, which is commonly associated with diabetes, predisposes to coronary atherosclerotic burden.[39] A small randomized trial of 33 subjects with INOCA found significant microvascular function improvement with metformin therapy, suggesting potential improvements of CMD in hyperglycemia reduction.[40]

Antiatherosclerotic Therapy

Aspirin
Aspirin inhibits platelet aggregation but also prevents the vasoconstrictive effects of thromboxane A2. The 2019 European Society of Cardiology guidelines for management of chronic coronary syndromes support at least one antiplatelet agent in diffuse epicardial atherosclerosis but in primary MVA, there is no robust evidence supporting a role of aspirin.[41]

Statin therapy
Statins are associated with anti-inflammatory and antiatherosclerotic effects.[9] Atorvastatin has been demonstrated to improve CFR in patients with slow coronary flow.[42] The 2019 European Society of Cardiology guidelines for management of chronic coronary syndromes suggest using statins in those with MVA.[41]

Angiotensin converting enzyme inhibitors (and angiotensin receptor blockade)
Angiotensin converting enzyme inhibitors act to block the vasoconstrictive effects of angiotensin II, which can reduce vascular tone and promote vasodilation.[23] In a randomized trial on 78 women with confirmed CMD, quinapril therapy was associated with reduction in angina frequency as well as improved CFR in invasive testing.[43] Combination therapy of ramipril and atorvastatin added to diltiazem in a randomized trial with 45 patients was shown to reduce frequency of angina in patients with CSX, suggesting likely some benefit in the CMD population, although CMD was not confirmed.[44]

Antianginal Therapy

Beta-blockers
Beta-blockers reduce myocardial oxygen demand and prolong diastolic filling, improving the chance of coronary flow meeting demand.[9,18] There are limited trials of beta-blocker use in patients with proven CMD. A comparison trial between propranolol and verapamil investigated 16 patients with angina and normal coronary arteries on angiography but no confirmed CMD. It found a significant reduction in angina in the beta-blocker arm compared with placebo but not in verapamil suggesting beta-blockers were superior to calcium channel blockade in this population.[45] A small 10 patient trial comparing atenolol, amlodipine, and nitrate therapy in CSX, showed angina improvement in the beta-blocker population but not in the nitrate or calcium channel blocker (CCB) populations.[46] Beta-blockers are recommended for MVA in the 2019 European Society of Cardiology guidelines for the management of chronic coronary syndromes.[41]

Nitrates
Nitrates act on arteriolar endothelium to cause vasodilation. Although traditionally prescribed for angina, accumulating evidence seem to suggest negligible benefit and even potential harm with the use of long-acting nitrates on MVA.[47,48] Reduced responsiveness from coronary arteries, steal syndrome from redistribution of blood flow to areas of adequate perfusion, and poor medication tolerance and have all been suggested as potential reasons for the lack of nitrate benefit in MVA.[47,48]

Calcium channel blockers
Calcium channel blockers act to cause coronary vasodilation and are particularly effective in

coronary vasospasm.[25] Limited trial benefit exists in CMD and diltiazem has been shown to not improve CFR in MVA.[9,49] Verapamil and Nifedipine use have been shown to improve angina symptoms in patients with angina and normal angiographic coronary arteries but this did not remove patients with vasospastic angina.[50] CCB are recommended after beta-blockers in patients with MVA according to 2013 ESC guidelines.[21]

Percutaneous coronary intervention Addressing epicardial coronary obstruction of significant lesions with percutaneous coronary intervention (PCI) when coexistent pathologic conditions exists may be important in the overall management of CMD. PCI should only be performed on physiologically significant stenosis (>90% or lesions with significant Fractional Flow Reserve (FFR) or Non-Hyperemia Pressure Ratio (NHPR).[21] Invasive physiological vessel interrogation allows appraisal of each coronary compartment and may predict improvement in epicardial blood flow after PCI of a coronary stenosis.[47,51] Invasive coronary physiology predicts ischemia relief but is less predictive of angina reduction.[52]

Novel Therapies

Ranolazine
Ranolazine improves myocardial perfusion by decreasing sodium and calcium overload through late sodium channel blockade, promoting myocardial relaxation.[23] Multiple mixed trial results exist where small benefits in CFR have been demonstrated,[53] as well as no benefit in others but benefit in angina symptoms.[54] Therefore, ranolazine requires larger trials to study its benefits.

Ivabradine
Ivabradine reduces heart rate thought I_f channel inhibition at the sinoatrial node. A small trial of 46 patients found symptomatic improvement of angina in ivabradine but no change in microvascular function.[54]

Phosphodiesterase inhibition
Sildenafil has been shown to improve CFR in women with CMD with the significant improvement being in those with a CFR of less than 2.5 but this was not clinically correlated with angina severity.[55]

Rho-kinase inhibition (fasudil)
Endothelin A receptor activates rho-kinase, eventually leading to vasoconstriction. Intracoronary fasudil, a rho-kinase inhibitor, improved angina and features of coronary ischemia in endothelin-dependent CMD.[56]

Zibotentan
Zibotentan is an endothelin A receptor antagonist, preventing the coronary vasoconstrictive effects of endothelin 1, which is often elevated in those with MVA.[57] It is currently undergoing phase 2 trials into its effect on exercise tolerance in MVA.[57]

Coronary sinus occlusion Coronary sinus occlusion can encourage retro filling of blood into the coronary microcirculation.[58,59] One such pressure-controlled intermittent coronary sinus occlusion device has been shown in the ST elevation myocardial infarction population to preserve microvascular function.[58] Another device to narrow the coronary sinus improved symptoms and quality of life in patients with refractory angina who were not candidates for revascularization.[59]

Spinal cord stimulation Electrical stimulation is thought to modulate pain fibers and possibly alter coronary blood flow. A small trial with 8 patients found small benefits in angina frequency in CSX with the use of transcutaneous electrical nerve stimulation.[60] Spinal cord stimulation has been demonstrated in a small trial of 7 subjects to improve angina and exercise tolerance in INOCA patients.[61]

Tricyclic antidepressants (imipramine, amitriptyline)
Tricyclic antidepressants aim to reduce nociceptive stimuli leading to reduced angina severity.[47] TCA's may have a role in treatment resistant MVA where enhanced pain perception is thought to possibly occur.

Hormone replacement Given the predisposition in the postmenopausal women population, estrogen deficiency has been suggested as a cause to CMD.[9] A small trial of 35 women demonstrated a reduction in angina symptoms in postmenopausal women and INOCA but did not alter endothelial dysfunction.[62]

Cognitive behavioral therapy CMD is often associated with anxiety and mood disorders. Autogenic relaxation training in 53 women demonstrated improvements in symptom frequency with CSX.[63] A small systemic review of 6 trials suggested a modest benefit predominately in the first 3 months of psychotherapy in individuals with chest pain and normal coronary arteries mainly focusing on cognitive behavioral framework. However, these patients had no formal CMD diagnosis made, and their pathogenesis could be broad (**Fig. 3**).

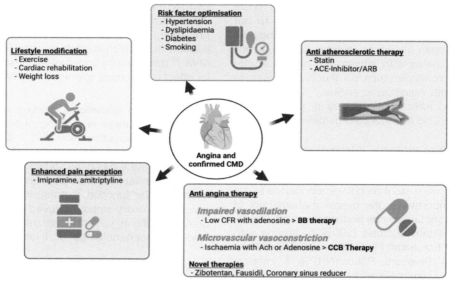

Fig. 3. Management of CMD principles.

SUMMARY

CMD remains a challenging condition to manage due to heterogenous pathophysiology, presentation, and response to therapy. Awareness of CMD is improving but therapeutic randomized trials of therapy are lacking. Invasive assessment of the coronary microcirculation can stratify anti-ischemic therapy to improved patient-centered outcomes. Beta-blockers remain the cornerstone of therapy for angina due to CMD. The role of non-pharmacological interventions including cardiovascular risk factor modification, lifestyle interventions, and cardiac rehabilitation is central to management. Further research is needed to assess traditional and novel pharmacological therapies on symptoms and clinical events in the various CMD endotypes.

CLINICS CARE POINTS

- Functional coronary angiography (coronary provocation testing) may be used to confirm the diagnosis of microvascular angina and tailor patient management.[26]

- Patients with microvascular angina and impaired vasodilator capacity (e.g. low CFR) may benefit from beta blocker therapy. This is the cornerstone of anti-ischaemic therapy in confirmed microvascular angina.[38,42,43]

- Increased microvascular constriction (e.g. microvascular spasm to acetylcholine infusion) often co-exists with epicardial coronary spasm and should be treated with calcium channel blockade.[21,47]

- Lifestyle modification is essential in managing CMD and should be implemented in all cases including smoking cessation, regular exercise, optimisation of diet and cardiac rehabilitation.[33, 62, 63]

- Hypertension, dyslipidaemia, and diabetes mellitus should all be treated to target as per standard primary prevention guidelines.[30,32,37]

- Statin and ACE Inhibitors are 'disease modifying therapies' for coronary atherosclerosis and may be beneficial in CMD.[41,39,38]

- Novel therapies targeting CMD are being explored in clinical trials including Zybotentan (endothelin A receptor inhibitor[54]).

- Subgroups of INOCA patients with enhanced nociception, altered pain pathways and/or associated depression may benefit from tricyclic antidepressants (amitriptyline 10 mg).[44]

DISCLOSURES

- T.J. Ford: Consultant/speaker/honorarium from Abbott Vascular, Boston Scientific, Boehringer Ingelheim, Biotronik, Bio-Excel, and Novartis.
- All other authors have no relevant disclosures. Funding was not required for the completion of this article.

REFERENCES

1. Khan MA, Hashim MJ, Mustafa H, et al. Global epidemiology of ischemic heart disease: results from the global burden of disease study. Cureus 2020;12(7):e9349.

2. Herscovici R, Sedlak T, Wei J, et al. Ischemia and no obstructive coronary artery disease (INOCA): what is the risk? J Am Heart Assoc 2018;7(17):e008868.

3. Vancheri F, Longo G, Vancheri S, et al. Coronary microvascular dysfunction. J Clin Med 2020;9(9): 1–36.

4. Lanza GA. Cardiac syndrome X: a critical overview and future perspectives. Heart 2007;93(2):159–66.

5. Beltrame JF, Tavella R, Jones D, et al. Management of ischaemia with non-obstructive coronary arteries (INOCA). BMJ 2021;375:e060602.

6. Ouellette ML, Löffler AI, Beller GA, et al. Clinical characteristics, sex differences, and outcomes in patients with normal or near-normal coronary arteries, non-obstructive or obstructive coronary artery disease. J Am Heart Assoc 2018;7(10):1–13.

7. Patel MR, Peterson ED, Dai D, et al. Low diagnostic yield of elective coronary angiography. N Engl J Med 2010;362(10):886–95.

8. Sara JD, Widmer RJ, Matsuzawa Y, et al. Prevalence of coronary microvascular dysfunction among patients with chest pain and nonobstructive coronary artery disease. JACC Cardiovasc Interv 2015; 8(11):1445–53.

9. Marinescu MA, Löffler AI, Ouellette M, et al. Coronary microvascular dysfunction, microvascular angina, and treatment strategies. JACC Cardiovasc Imaging 2015;8(2):210–20.

10. Ford TJ, Yii E, Sidik N, et al. Ischemia and no obstructive coronary artery disease: prevalence and correlates of coronary vasomotion disorders. Circ Cardiovasc interventions 2019;12(12):e008126.

11. Bugiardini R, Bairey Merz CN. Angina with "normal" coronary arteries: a changing philosophy. JAMA 2005;293(4):477–84.

12. Aribas E, van Lennep JER, Elias-Smale SE, et al. Prevalence of microvascular angina among patients with stable symptoms in the absence of obstructive coronary artery disease: a systematic review. Cardiovasc Res 2021;118(3):763–71.

13. Ong P, Camici PG, Beltrame JF, et al. International standardization of diagnostic criteria for microvascular angina. Int J Cardiol 2018;250:16–20.

14. Jespersen L, Hvelplund A, Abildstrøm SZ, et al. Stable angina pectoris with no obstructive coronary artery disease is associated with increased risks of major adverse cardiovascular events. Eur Heart J 2012;33(6):734–44.

15. Jespersen L, Abildstrøm SZ, Hvelplund A, et al. Persistent angina: highly prevalent and associated with long-term anxiety, depression, low physical functioning, and quality of life in stable angina pectoris. Clin Res Cardiol 2013;102(8):571–81.

16. Shimokawa H, Suda A, Takahashi J, et al. Clinical characteristics and prognosis of patients with microvascular angina: an international and prospective cohort study by the Coronary Vasomotor Disorders International Study (COVADIS) Group. Eur Heart J 2021;42(44):4592–600.

17. Bairey Merz CN, Pepine CJ, Shimokawa H, et al. Treatment of coronary microvascular dysfunction. Cardiovasc Res 2020;116(4):856–70.

18. Chen C, Wei J, AlBadri A, et al. Coronary microvascular dysfunction - epidemiology, pathogenesis, prognosis, diagnosis, risk factors and therapy. Circ J 2016;81(1):3–11.

19. Camici PG, Crea F. Coronary microvascular dysfunction. N Engl J Med 2007;356(8):830–40.

20. Kuruvilla S, Kramer CM. Coronary microvascular dysfunction in women: an overview of diagnostic strategies. Expert Rev Cardiovasc Ther 2013; 11(11):1515–25.

21. Montalescot G, Sechtem U, Achenbach S, et al. 2013 ESC guidelines on the management of stable coronary artery disease: the Task Force on the management of stable coronary artery disease of the European Society of Cardiology. Eur Heart J 2013; 34(38):2949–3003.

22. Gdowski MA, Murthy VL, Doering M, et al. Association of isolated coronary microvascular dysfunction with mortality and major adverse cardiac events: a systematic review and meta-analysis of aggregate data. J Am Heart Assoc 2020;9(9):e014954.

23. Taqueti VR, Di Carli MF. Coronary microvascular disease pathogenic mechanisms and therapeutic options: JACC state-of-the-art review. J Am Coll Cardiol 2018;72(21):2625–41.

24. Shaw J, Anderson T. Coronary endothelial dysfunction in non-obstructive coronary artery disease: risk, pathogenesis, diagnosis and therapy. Vasc Med 2016;21(2):146–55.

25. McIvor ME, Undemir C, Lawson J, et al. Clinical effects and utility of intracoronary diltiazem. Cathet Cardiovasc Diagn 1995;35(4):287–91 [discussion: 292-283].

26. Ford TJ, Stanley B, Sidik N, et al. 1-Year outcomes of angina management guided by invasive coronary function testing (CorMicA). JACC Cardiovasc Interv 2020;13(1):33–45.

27. Ghisi GL, Abdallah F, Grace SL, et al. A systematic review of patient education in cardiac patients: do they increase knowledge and promote health behavior change? Patient Educ Couns 2014;95(2): 160–74.

28. den Hollander M, de Jong JR, Volders S, et al. Fear reduction in patients with chronic pain: a learning theory perspective. Expert Rev Neurother 2010; 10(11):1733–45.

29. Beck EB, Erbs S, Möbius-Winkler S, et al. Exercise training restores the endothelial response to vascular growth factors in patients with stable coronary artery disease. Eur J Prev Cardiol 2012;19(3): 412–8.

30. Czernin J, Barnard RJ, Sun KT, et al. Effect of short-term cardiovascular conditioning and low-fat diet on myocardial blood flow and flow reserve. Circulation 1995;92(2):197–204.

31. Kissel CK, Nikoletou D. Cardiac rehabilitation and exercise prescription in symptomatic patients with non-obstructive coronary artery disease-a systematic review. Curr Treat Options Cardiovasc Med 2018;20(9):78.

32. Mizuno R, Fujimoto S, Saito Y, et al. Optimal antihypertensive level for improvement of coronary microvascular dysfunction: the lower, the better? Hypertension 2012;60(2):326–32.

33. Schwartzkopff B, Brehm M, Mundhenke M, et al. Repair of coronary arterioles after treatment with perindopril in hypertensive heart disease. Hypertension 2000;36(2):220–5.

34. Dayanikli F, Grambow D, Muzik O, et al. Early detection of abnormal coronary flow reserve in asymptomatic men at high risk for coronary artery disease using positron emission tomography. Circulation 1994;90(2):808–17.

35. Yokoyama I, Murakami T, Ohtake T, et al. Reduced coronary flow reserve in familial hypercholesterolemia. J Nucl Med 1996;37(12):1937–42.

36. Lee DH, Youn HJ, Choi YS, et al. Coronary flow reserve is a comprehensive indicator of cardiovascular risk factors in subjects with chest pain and normal coronary angiogram. Circ J 2010;74(7): 1405–14.

37. Kaufmann PA, Gnecchi-Ruscone T, di Terlizzi M, et al. Coronary heart disease in smokers: vitamin C restores coronary microcirculatory function. Circulation 2000;102(11):1233–8.

38. Di Carli MF, Janisse J, Grunberger G, et al. Role of chronic hyperglycemia in the pathogenesis of coronary microvascular dysfunction in diabetes. J Am Coll Cardiol 2003;41(8):1387–93.

39. Bettencourt N, Toschke AM, Leite D, et al. Epicardial adipose tissue is an independent predictor of coronary atherosclerotic burden. Int J Cardiol 2012; 158(1):26–32.

40. Jadhav S, Ferrell W, Greer IA, et al. Effects of metformin on microvascular function and exercise tolerance in women with angina and normal coronary arteries: a randomized, double-blind, placebo-controlled study. J Am Coll Cardiol 2006;48(5): 956–63.

41. Knuuti J, Wijns W, Saraste A, et al. 2019 ESC Guidelines for the diagnosis and management of chronic coronary syndromes. Eur Heart J 2020;41(3): 407–77.

42. Caliskan M, Erdogan D, Gullu H, et al. Effects of atorvastatin on coronary flow reserve in patients with slow coronary flow. Clin Cardiol 2007;30(9):475–9.

43. Pauly DF, Johnson BD, Anderson RD, et al. In women with symptoms of cardiac ischemia, nonobstructive coronary arteries, and microvascular dysfunction, angiotensin-converting enzyme inhibition is associated with improved microvascular function: a double-blind randomized study from the National Heart, Lung and Blood Institute Women's Ischemia Syndrome Evaluation (WISE). Am Heart J 2011;162(4):678–84.

44. Pizzi C, Manfrini O, Fontana F, et al. Angiotensin-converting enzyme inhibitors and 3-hydroxy-3-methylglutaryl coenzyme A reductase in cardiac Syndrome X: role of superoxide dismutase activity. Circulation 2004;109(1):53–8.

45. Bugiardini R, Borghi A, Biagetti L, et al. Comparison of verapamil versus propranolol therapy in syndrome X. Am J Cardiol 1989;63(5):286–90.

46. Lanza GA, Colonna G, Pasceri V, et al. Atenolol versus amlodipine versus isosorbide-5-mononitrate on anginal symptoms in syndrome X. Am J Cardiol 1999;84(7):854–6. a858.

47. Ford TJ, Berry C. Angina: contemporary diagnosis and management. Heart 2020;106(5):387–98.

48. Beltrame JF, Horowitz JD. Why do nitrates have limited efficacy in coronary microvessels?: Editorial to: "Lack of nitrates on exercise stress test results in patients with microvascular angina" by G. Russo et al. Cardiovasc Drugs Ther 2013;27(3):187–8.

49. Sütsch G, Oechslin E, Mayer I, et al. Effect of diltiazem on coronary flow reserve in patients with microvascular angina. Int J Cardiol 1995;52(2): 135–43.

50. Cannon RO 3rd, Watson RM, Rosing DR, et al. Efficacy of calcium channel blocker therapy for angina pectoris resulting from small-vessel coronary artery disease and abnormal vasodilator reserve. Am J Cardiol 1985;56(4):242–6.

51. Ford TJ, Berry C, De Bruyne B, et al. Physiological predictors of acute coronary syndromes: emerging insights from the plaque to the vulnerable patient. JACC Cardiovasc interventions 2017;10(24): 2539–47.

52. Al-Lamee R, Howard JP, Shun-Shin MJ, et al. Fractional flow reserve and instantaneous wave-free ratio as predictors of the placebo-controlled response to percutaneous coronary intervention in stable single-vessel coronary artery disease: physiology-stratified analysis of ORBITA. Circulation 2018;138(17): 1780–92.

53. Mehta PK, Goykhman P, Thomson LE, et al. Ranolazine improves angina in women with evidence of myocardial ischemia but no obstructive coronary artery disease. JACC Cardiovasc Imaging 2011;4(5): 514–22.

54. Villano A, Di Franco A, Nerla R, et al. Effects of ivabradine and ranolazine in patients with microvascular angina pectoris. Am J Cardiol 2013;112(1):8–13.

55. Denardo SJ, Wen X, Handberg EM, et al. Effect of phosphodiesterase type 5 inhibition on microvascular coronary dysfunction in women: a Women's Ischemia Syndrome Evaluation (WISE) ancillary study. Clin Cardiol 2011;34(8):483–7.

56. Mohri M, Shimokawa H, Hirakawa Y, et al. Rho-kinase inhibition with intracoronary fasudil prevents myocardial ischemia in patients with coronary microvascular spasm. J Am Coll Cardiol 2003;41(1):15–9.

57. Morrow AJ, Ford TJ, Mangion K, et al. Rationale and design of the Medical Research Council's Precision Medicine with Zibotentan in Microvascular Angina (PRIZE) trial. Am Heart J 2020;229:70–80.

58. Scarsini R, Terentes-Printzios D, Shanmuganathan M, et al. Pressure-controlled intermittent coronary sinus occlusion improves the vasodilatory microvascular capacity and reduces myocardial injury in patients with STEMI. Catheter Cardiovasc Interv 2021;99(2): 329–39.

59. Verheye S, Jolicœur EM, Behan MW, et al. Efficacy of a device to narrow the coronary sinus in refractory angina. N Engl J Med 2015;372(6):519–27.

60. Jessurun GA, Hautvast RW, Tio RA, et al. Electrical neuromodulation improves myocardial perfusion and ameliorates refractory angina pectoris in patients with syndrome X: fad or future? Eur J Pain 2003;7(6):507–12.

61. Lanza GA, Sestito A, Sandric S, et al. Spinal cord stimulation in patients with refractory anginal pain and normal coronary arteries. Ital Heart J 2001; 2(1):25–30.

62. Merz CN, Olson MB, McClure C, et al. A randomized controlled trial of low-dose hormone therapy on myocardial ischemia in postmenopausal women with no obstructive coronary artery disease: results from the National Institutes of Health/National Heart, Lung, and Blood Institute-sponsored Women's Ischemia Syndrome Evaluation (WISE). Am Heart J 2010;159(6). 987.e981-987.

63. Asbury EA, Kanji N, Ernst E, et al. Autogenic training to manage symptomology in women with chest pain and normal coronary arteries. Menopause 2009; 16(1):60–5.

The Ability of Near-Infrared Spectroscopy to Identify Vulnerable Patients and Plaques: A Systematic Review and Meta-Analysis

Ronald D. Bass, BA[a], Joseph Phillips, BS, MS[b],
Jorge Sanz Sánchez, MD, PhD[c,d], Priti Shah, MSc[e], Stephen Sum, PhD[e],
Ron Waksman, MD[f], Hector M. Garcia-Garcia, MD, PhD[f,*]

KEYWORDS

- NIRS • Vulnerable plaque • ACS • LRP

KEY POINTS

- A near-infrared spectroscopy (NIRS) meta-analysis provides a more precise estimate of the efficacy of NIRS.
- NIRS-derived lipid core burden index (LCBI) is an effective method for quantifying and identifying high-risk plaques and patients at increased risk of future MACE/MACCE.
- A maxLCBI$_{4mm}$ of 400 or greater seems to be an effective threshold for classifying at-risk plaques.

INTRODUCTION

Coronary artery disease continues to be a major cause of global morbidity and mortality despite medical advancements and effective preventive measures.[1] Acute coronary syndromes (ACS) are most often caused by rupture or fissure of a lipid-rich core-containing plaque and a large plaque burden, termed a vulnerable plaque.[2,3] Autopsy findings determined that these atheromas have a large plaque size, cholesterol-rich lipid core, and thin fibrous cap.[4] Atheromas tend to occur at multiple sites resulting in high atherosclerotic burden, which confers to a patient at high-risk of adverse cardiac events.[2] More recently, research has focused on preemptively identifying at-risk plaques and patients in a more proactive strategy of targeted secondary prevention.

Currently, the only imaging modality validated to identify lipid-rich plaques is near-infrared spectroscopy (NIRS).[5] NIRS uses unique technology via an add-on optic fiber as part of an imaging system attached to an intravascular ultrasound (IVUS) catheter that can easily identify lipid-rich plaque.[5] NIRS is able to deliver quantitative data regarding lipid composition within coronary artery walls, providing a more precise identification of vulnerable plaques than previously available,[6] which may provide clinicians with improved patient-level risk estimation for more targeted interventions.

Although NIRS has been evaluated in the context of many different clinical scenarios, for

This article originally appeared in *Interventional Cardiology Clinics*, Volume 12, Issue 2, January 2023.
ᵃ School of Medicine, Georgetown University, 3800 Reservoir Road, NorthWest, Washington, DC 20007, USA; ᵇ University of Iowa Hospitals and Clinics, 200 Hawkins Drive Iowa City, IA 52242, USA; ᶜ Hospital Universitari I Politecnic La Fe, Avinguda de Fernando Abril Martorell, no 106, 46026 València, Spain; ᵈ Centro de Investigación Biomedica en Red (CIBERCV), Avenue, Monforte de Lemos, 3-5. Pabellón 11. Planta 0. 28029 Madrid, Spain; ᵉ InfraRedx, A Nipro Company, 28 Crosby Drive, Suite 100, Bedford, MA 01730, USA; ᶠ Interventional Cardiology, MedStar Washington Hospital Center, 110 Irving Street, 4B-1, Washington, DC, 20010, USA
* Corresponding author. 110 Irving Street, Suite 4B-1, Washington, DC, 20010,
E-mail addresses: hector.m.garciagarcia@medstar.net; hect2701@gmail.com

the purposes of this study, we chose to focus on the association of NIRS and cardiovascular (CV) outcomes. Emerging evidence suggest that NIRS-derived lipid core burden index (LCBI) provides prognostic data at the patient level as well as the plaque level. Individual studies evaluating the role of NIRS are characterized by the inclusion of a small number of patients and may not provide adequately powered analysis, thus prompting the need for a systematic appraisal of treatment effects and quality of evidence. Therefore, this systematic review and meta-analysis aims to compile the currently available data regarding the prognostic value of NIRS-derived LCBI on adverse cardiac outcomes to provide more precise effect estimates.

METHODS
Protocol

This systematic review and meta-analysis was performed according to the Preferred Reporting Items for Systematic Reviews and Meta-Analyses (PRISMA) reporting guidelines.[7] The corresponding author had full access to all the data and had final responsibility for the decision to submit for publication. The data supporting the findings in this study are available from the corresponding author on reasonable request.

Search Strategy

We performed a comprehensive literature search of all published studies—retrospective, prospective, observational—available through PubMed and Ovid (inception through December 31, 2021), without language restrictions. Case reports, letters to the editor, reviews, and book chapters were not included in this meta-analysis. Key search terms used were, "NIRS," "IVUS," "LCBI," "MACE," "MACCE," "coronary artery disease," "coronary heart disease," "angina," "myocardial infarction," "acute myocardial infarct," "myocardial ischemia," "acute coronary syndrome," "ischemic heart disease" including their subheadings, MeSH terms, and all synonyms. References for each of the studies selected were also screened. The PRISMA guidelines were applied for this search process.

Selection Criteria

Studies were eligible if they met the following criteria: (1) investigated the diagnostic performance of NIRS in predicting adverse cardiac outcomes; (2) in a patient population undergoing an invasive catheterization laboratory procedure, regardless of indication; (3) involving a unique patient population not included in another study; and

(4) reported at least 1 of the following CV outcomes: all-cause mortality, CV mortality, myocardial infarction, stroke, or urgent coronary revascularization. Study selection was performed by 2 independent reviewers (R.B. and J.P.), first by screening of titles and abstracts, followed by review of full texts and their corresponding references. In cases in which there was a disagreement over eligibility, a third reviewer (H.G.) assessed the discrepancy, and decisions were reached by consensus. Quality of the data was analyzed using the Downs and Black Checklist or the Cochrane Risk of Bias tools, as applicable, by study type. An overview of referenced studies is provided in **Table 1**.

Data Extraction

Data on study characteristics, patient characteristics, and endpoint event rates were independently extracted and organized into a structured data set by 2 reviewers (R.B. and J.P.), compared, and reported in **Table 2**. Any discrepancy resulted in reevaluation of the primary data and involvement of a third reviewer (H.G.), with disagreements resolved by consensus.

Outcomes of Interest

The central illustration (**Fig. 1**) shows an example of a NIRS-derived chemogram and the value of NIRS in identifying high-risk patients and plaques. The prespecified primary endpoint in this study was major adverse cardiovascular and cerebrovascular events (MACCE). For trials not reporting MACCE, MACE was chosen as primary endpoint.[8–14] Note that $maxLCBI_{4mm}$ was used in all studies except Danek and colleagues, which did not have the data available, and therefore used the LCBI of the vessel with highest lipid burden.[10] Thus, the authors of this article use the term LCBI to refer to all the NIRS-derived measurements for purposes of the primary analysis. Note that the $maxLCBI_{4mm}$ refers to the 4 mm long segment with the maximum LCBI. The authors of this study then investigated their own secondary endpoint using a threshold $maxLCBI_{4mm}$ at or around 400 as suggested by prior studies including Waksman and colleagues.[13] Each endpoint was assessed according to the definitions reported in the original study protocols. The list of endpoints for each study is listed in **Table 3** along with the definitions of each endpoint.

Risk of Bias

Methodological quality of included studies was assessed using the Risk of Bias In Nonrandomized Studies of Interventions assessment

Table 1
Study overviews

Trial/Author Year	Study Design	Multicenter	Population	Follow-Up
Oemrawsingh, et al,[8] 2014	Observational (prospective) Primary endpoint: MACCE	No	Patients with clinical indication for diagnostic coronary angiography and/or PCI due to ACS or stable CAD	1 y
Madder, et al,[9] 2016	Observational (prospective) Primary endpoint: MACCE	No	Patients with clinical indication for invasive coronary angiography and/or PCI due to ACS or stable CAD	1.7 y ± 0.4 y
Danek, et al,[10] 2017	Observational (prospective) Primary endpoint: MACE	No	Patients with clinically indicated cardiac catheterization and NIRS imaging due to ACS or stable CAD	Median 5.3 y
Schuurman, et al,[11] 2017	Observational (prospective) Primary endpoint: MACE	No	Patients undergoing diagnostic coronary angiography or PCI due to ACS or stable CAD	Median 4.1 y
Karlsson, et al,[12] 2019	Observational (retrospective enrollment, prospective follow-up) Primary endpoint: MACCE	Yes	Patients with clinical indication for coronary catheterization due to ACS or stable CAD	Mean 2.9 ± 1.3 y
LRP Study Waksman, et al,[13] 2019	Prospective, cohort Primary endpoint: MACE	Yes	Patients with indication for cardiac catheterization with possible ad hoc PCI due to known or suspected ACS or stable CAD	2 y
PROSPECT II Erlinge, et al,[14] 2021	Prospective, observational Primary endpoint: MACE	Yes	Patients intended for coronary angiography ± PCI due to recent STEMI or NSTEMI enrolled after successful intervention of all flow-limiting culprit lesions	Median 3.7 y

Abbreviations: CAD, coronary artery disease; NSTEMI, non-ST segment elevation myocardial infarction; PCI, percutaneous coronary intervention; STEMI, ST segment elevation myocardial infarction.

Table 2
Background characteristics

Trial/Author	Age[b] (y)	Men (%)	HTN (%)	DM2 (%)	HLD (%)	Prior MI (%)	Prior PCI (%)	Prior CABG (%)	Prior Stroke (%)	Index Presentation (%)
Oemrawsingh, et al,[8] 2014	63.4	72.9	56.2	20.2	56.7	38.9	38.4	3.0	3.0	Composite ACS 46.8 Stable Symptoms 53.2
Madder, et al,[9] 2016	62.5	68.6	57.9	19.8	57.9	14.0	18.2	NR	5.0	Composite ACS 85.1 Stable Symptoms 14.9
Danek, et al,[10] 2017[a]	63.5	99	95	50	93	36	11	23	11.0	Composite ACS 39 Stable Symptoms 61
Schuurman, et al,[11] 2017	62.5	76.7	60.0	21.5	57.5	34.2	35.6	2.2	5.8	Composite ACS 42.5 Stable Symptoms 57.5
Karlsson, et al,[12] 2019	66.5	70.8	53.5	19.4	NR	29.2	NR	NR	9.7	Composite ACS 81.9 Stable Symptoms 18.1
LRP Study (Waksman, et al,[13] 2019)	64.0	69.5	80.4	36.7	80.3	23.5	44.9	NR	NR	Composite ACS 53.7 Stable Symptoms 46.3
PROSPECT II (Erlinge, et al,[14] 2021)	63.0	83.0	37.2[c]	12.1	25.2[d]	9.9	11.9	0.0	5.2	Composite ACS 100.0

Included background characteristics refer to the full study populations as defined in **Table 1** of the individual studies.
Abbreviations: CABG, coronary artery bypass graft; CAD, coronary artery disease; DM2, diabetes mellitus type 2; HLD, hyperlipidemia; HTN, hypertension; MI, myocardial infarction; NSTEMI, non-ST segment elevation MI; PCI, percutaneous coronary intervention; SAP, stable angina pectoris; STEMI, ST segment elevation MI; Sx, symptoms; UAP, unstable angina pectoris.
[a] Authors did not present any decimals.
[b] All ages are reported as means except Erlinge et al. is a median.
[c] HTN in PROSPECT-II defined as hypertension requiring medication.
[d] HLD in PROSPECT-II defined as hyperlipidemia requiring medication.

Tool from Cochrane handbook (ROBINS-I). Two investigators (R.B. and J.P) independently assessed 7 domains of bias: (1) confounding, (2) selection of participants, (3) classification of interventions, (4) deviations from intended interventions, (5) missing outcome data, (6) measurement of the outcome, and (7) selection of the reported results.

Statistical Analysis

Odds ratios (OR) and 95% confidence intervals (CI) were calculated using the DerSimonian and Laird random-effects model, with the estimate of heterogeneity being taken from the Mantel-Haenszel method. When the required numbers to pool the data were not available in the text or tables, we used an online semiautomated software to extract underlying numerical data from applicable Kaplan-Meier curves provided to determine the number of events above and below the relevant LCBI threshold in each study (WebPlotDigitizer 4.5, Ankit Rohatgi, Pacifica, California, USA). The presence of heterogeneity among studies was evaluated with the Cochran Q chi-square test, with $P \leq .10$ considered of statistical significance, and using the I^2 test to evaluate

inconsistency. A value of 0% indicates no observed heterogeneity, and larger values indicate increasing heterogeneity. I^2 values of 25% or lesser, 50% or lesser, and greater than 50% indicated low, moderate, and high heterogeneity, respectively. A prespecified sensitivity analyses was performed by removing the studies not using a threshold maxLCBI$_{4mm}$ at or around 400.

Analyses were performed according to the intention-to-treat principle. The statistical level of significance was 2-tailed $P < .05$. Statistical analyses were performed with the Stata software version 13.1 (StataCorp LP, College Station, Texas, USA).

RESULTS
Search Results

A total of 7 studies involving 2948 patients were identified for this study as shown in **Table 1**. Each study was published within the last 10 years. All were observational studies with prospective follow-up.

Two of the studies, Schuurman and colleagues and Oemrawsingh and colleagues, included the same study population with results reported at different periods of follow-up.[8,11] Because

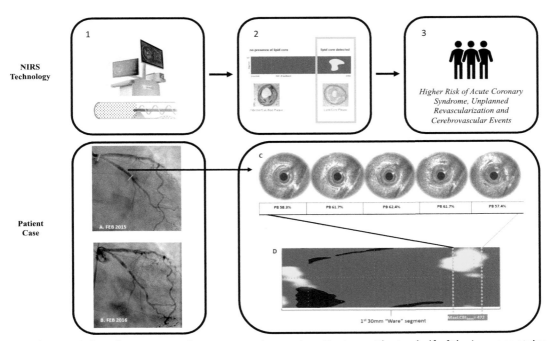

Fig. 1. The near-infrared spectroscopy instrument and example patient case. The top half of the image contains 3 panels, labeled 1 to 3 and outlined with black boxes, to introduce the near-infrared spectroscopy technology. The top image in panel 1 shows the NIRS machine while the bottom image in panel 1 shows the Dualpro catheter that delivers light to the vessel wall. Panel 2 is an example chemogram derived from the machine in panel 1. The red and yellow colors differentiate plaque characteristics. Yellow color on the chemogram as shown represents lipid core plaque. There is a yellow box around the identified lipid core plaque. Panel 3 emphasizes the association of this type of lipid core plaque with patient morbidity and mortality, particularly events defined in MACE/MACCE such as acute coronary syndrome, unplanned coronary revascularization, and cerebrovascular events. The bottom half of the figure shows a patient case representing the utility of NIRS.[13] There are 2 parts outlined with black boxes, each with 2 panels, labeled (A–D). Panel A shows the baseline coronary angiography of the left circumflex artery with no stenosis at the time of study enrollment. The light blue lines correspond to the 30 mm Ware segment as defined in the study protocol. Panel B shows the follow-up coronary angiography 1 year later, this time with a new significant lesion on the left circumflex. The intravascular ultrasound grayscale images in Panel C correspond to the maxLCBI$_{4mm}$ at baseline. The plaque burden of each 1-mm interval frame is found underneath each intravascular ultrasound image. In each interval, the plaque burden is moderate, between 57.4% and 62.4%. (A) NIRS-derived chemogram of the 30 mm Ware segment at baseline is seen in Panel D, indicating a maxLCBI$_{4mm}$ of 472. This patient case emphasizes the importance of NIRS-identification of lipid-rich plaque. Even though the angiography at baseline showed no stenosis, the area with maxLCBI$_{4mm}$ as discovered by NIRS was the culprit of a new lesion 1 year later. NIRS can predict potential areas of complication and provide an opportunity for prevention at the patient and plaque level.

Schuurman and colleagues published results with a greater duration of follow-up and larger sample size the authors chose to include those results and exclude Oemrawsingh and colleagues from the statistical analysis. Furthermore, although the total study population in Danek and colleagues was 239 patients, available data for nontarget vessel LCBI was only available for 39 patients.

Baseline Characteristics

Main baseline characteristics of included patients for each individual study are summarized in **Table 2**. Most patients were men with a mean age ranging from 62.5 to 66.5 years. The percentage

of patients with hypertension ranged between 37.2% and 95%, whereas those with type 2 diabetes ranged from 12.1% to 50%. The presence of hyperlipidemia was between 25.2% and 93%. A subset of patients in each study experienced prior myocardial infarction, ranging from 9.9% to 38.9% of the populations. ACS was the index presentation in between 39% and 100% of patients.

Clinical Outcomes

The primary analysis and individual OR are shown in **Fig. 2**. The 6 included studies used different LCBI thresholds, ranging from LCBI of 77 or

Table 3
Outcome definitions

Trial/Author	MACCE	MACE	ACS	Cerebrovascular Events	MI	Unstable Angina	Unplanned Coronary Revascularization	Cardiac Death
Oemrawsingh, et al,[8] 2014	All-cause mortality Nonfatal ACS Stroke Unplanned coronary revascularization	NR	Per guidelines of the European Society of Cardiology	Per guidelines of the European Stroke Organization	NR	NR	PCI or CABG which initially was not planned after index angiography and study enrollment	NR
Madder, et al,[9] 2016	All-cause mortality Nonfatal ACS Acute cerebrovascular events	NR	MI or UA arising from a de novo culprit lesion and requiring revascularization	TIA or stroke	Universal definition	ACS presentations in the absence of cardiac biomarker elevations	NR	NR
Danek, et al,[10] 2017	NR	Cardiac death ACS Unplanned coronary revascularization Stroke after discharge from index hospitalization	Third Universal Definition of Myocardial Infarction	NR	Third Universal Definition	Third Universal Definition	PCI or CABG that was not planned after the index coronary angiography and NIRS imaging procedure	NR
Schuurman, et al,[11] 2017	NR	All-cause death Non-fatal ACS Unplanned coronary revascularization	Per guidelines of the European Society of Cardiology	NR	ESC Guidelines	ESC Guidelines	Any PCI or CABG that was not planned after the index angiography and enrollment in the study	Any death due to proximate cardiac cause, unwitnessed death or death of unknown cause
Karlsson, et al,[12] 2019	All-cause mortality Recurrent ACS requiring revascularization Cerebrovascular events	NR	Event requiring revascularization	TIA or stroke	NR	NR	NR	NR

LRP Study (Waksman, et al,[13] 2019)	NR	Nonculprit cardiac death, cardiac arrest, nonfatal MI, ACS, revascularization by CABG or PCI, and readmission to hospital for angina with more than 20% diameter stenosis progression	UA or MI requiring revascularization as defined in PROSPECT I[19]	2014 ACC/AHA Definition (TIA or Stroke)	2014 ACC/AHA and PROSPECT I[19] Definition	NR	All interventional cardiology methods for treatment of coronary artery disease and 2014 ACC/AHA Definition	2014 ACC/AHA Definition: Any death due to immediate cardiac cause (MI, low-output failure, fatal arrhythmia)
PROSPECT II (Erlinge, et al,[14] 2021)	NR	Cardiac death MI Unstable angina Progressive angina either requiring revascularization or with rapid lesion progression (defined in the appendix) arising from untreated, nonculprit lesions during follow-up	NR	Intracranial hemorrhage or nonhemorrhagic stroke that led to death	Third Universal Definition and SCAI criteria	Ischemic chest pain (or equivalent) at rest considered to be myocardial ischemia on final diagnosis and without elevation in cardiac biomarkers of necrosis	NR	The composite of sudden cardiac death, death due to acute myocardial infarction, death due to heart failure, death due to arrhythmia, or death not due to known vascular or non-CV causes

Abbreviations: NR, not reported.

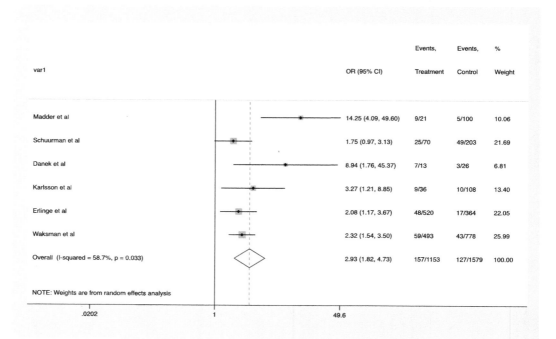

Fig. 2. Odds ratios and 95% confidence intervals for the occurrence of MACE/MACCE during follow-up after index presentation associated with all LCBI thresholds. The forest plot shows the results from the 6 included studies in the meta-analysis, listed by first author, along with the overall pooled summary estimate. The x-axis represents odds ratio values. The odds ratios and associated 95% confidence intervals are reported as a dot and line segment, respectively. The size of square data markers is proportional to the study weight in the meta-analysis. The summary measure point estimate and 95% confidence interval is represented as a diamond at the bottom of the plot. Number of events in the treatment group, defined as LCBI above threshold, and control group, defined as LCBI below threshold, used in the odds ratio calculations are provided on the right side of the table. All included study results suggest that LCBI values above the prespecified threshold was significantly associated with an increased odds of MACE/MACCE during follow-up. The thresholds used are as follows: $maxLCBI_{4mm} \geq 400$, $maxLCBI_{4mm} \geq 360$ (fourth quartile), $LCBI \geq 77$ (determined using receiver-operator characteristic analysis), $maxLCBI_{4mm} \geq 400$, $maxLCBI_{4mm} \geq 324.7$, and $maxLCBI_{4mm} > 400$ for Madder, Schuurman, Danek, Karlsson, Erlinge, and Waksman and colleagues, respectively.

greater to LCBI of 400 or greater (specifically, $maxLCBI_{4mm}$). Overall, identification of vulnerable plaques with NIRS is associated with 2.93 times increased odds of MACE/MACCE (95% CI 1.82–4.73, $I^2 = 58.7\%$) in the pooled meta-analysis. Waksman and colleagues was weighted the most at 25.99%. Erlinge and colleagues was weighted the second highest at 22.05%.

The secondary outcome is shown in **Fig. 3**, which provides a forest plot depicting pooled results from studies using a max 4 mm LCBI threshold at or around 400. Studies included for the secondary endpoint were Madder and colleagues, Schuurman and colleagues, Karlsson and colleagues, Erlinge and colleagues, and Waksman and colleagues. Madder and colleagues, Karlsson and colleagues, and Waksman and colleagues used 400 as the threshold $maxLCBI_{4mm}$. Schuurman and colleagues used

$maxLCBI_{4mm}$ of 360 or greater and Erlinge and colleagues used $maxLCBI_{4mm}$ of 324.7 or greater as the primary analysis, both representing the upper quartile. The pooled odds ratio was 2.67 (95% CI 1.67–4.25, $I^2 = 58.4\%$). Waksman and colleagues and Erlinge and colleagues again were weighted the most at 28.79% and 23.85%, respectively.

Risk of Bias Assessment

All included studies were considered at high overall risk of bias.

DISCUSSION
Meta-Analysis Findings

This quantitative analysis showed that the detection of large lipid-rich plaque by NIRS is a powerful tool to predict major adverse CV events in patients with coronary artery disease. The main

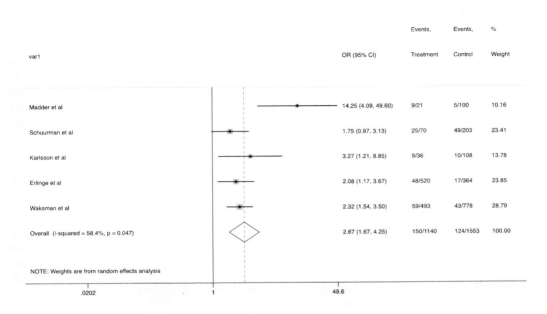

Fig. 3. Odds ratios and 95% confidence intervals for the occurrence of MACE/MACCE during follow-up after index presentation associated with maxLCBI$_{4mm}$ thresholds at or around 400. The forest plot shows the results from the 5 included studies in the meta-analysis, listed by first author, along with the overall pooled summary estimate. The x-axis represents odds ratio values. The odds ratios and associated 95% confidence intervals are reported as a dot and line segment, respectively. The size of square data markers is proportional to the study weight in the meta-analysis. The summary measure point estimate and 95% confidence interval is represented as a diamond at the bottom of the plot. Number of events in the treatment group, defined as maxLCBI$_{4mm}$ above threshold, and control group, defined as maxLCBI$_{4mm}$ below threshold, used in the odds ratio calculations are provided on the right side of the table. All included study results suggest that maxLCBI$_{4mm}$ values above the prespecified threshold was significantly associated with an increased odds of MACE/MACCE during follow-up. The thresholds used are as follows: maxLCBI$_{4mm} \geq$ 400, maxLCBI$_{4mm} \geq$ 360 (fourth quartile), maxLCBI$_{4mm} \geq$ 400, maxLCBI$_{4mm-} \geq$ 324.7, and maxLCBI$_{4mm} >$ 400 for Madder, Schuurman, Karlsson, Erlinge, and Waksman and colleagues, respectively.

contribution of this meta-analysis is the significantly improved precision of the pooled estimate odds ratio of 2.93 (95% CI 1.82–4.73) as seen in **Fig. 2**. The 95% CIs of the individual OR from each study were generally wider and more varied, with the narrowest interval of OR 1.54 to 3.50 in Waksman and colleagues and the widest interval of OR 1.76 to 45.37 in Danek and colleagues. The pooled estimate provides a narrow CI of OR 1.82 to 4.73. This more precise odds ratio with a narrow standard deviation of the relationship between lipid-rich plaques identified by NIRS and subsequent adverse events can be used in future studies to guide sample size calculations.

Furthermore, this meta-analysis confirms maxLCBI$_{4mm}$ of 400 or greater as an appropriate cutoff for identifying high-risk lipid rich plaques at the patient and individual plaque level. Similarly, it improves the precision of this cutoff in predicting

adverse events. The narrowest 95% CI of the 4 included studies was Waksman and colleagues from 1.54 to 3.50 while the widest interval was Madder and colleagues from 4.09 to 49.60. The pooled estimate from the meta-analysis provided an OR of 2.67 with a 95% CI of 1.67 to 4.25. This suggests that this is a reasonable binary cutoff to use in future studies.

Literature Review

Relationship between increasing lipid core burden index and adverse events

NIRS is a catheter-based intracoronary imaging technique that uses diffuse reflectance spectroscopy to measure the chemical signature of cholesterol within the coronary vessel wall. The specific molecular features of cholesterol lie within the near-infrared light wavelength region and can thus be distinguished from collagen to identify lipid-rich plaques from normal vessel or fibrotic and calcified plaques.[8] The technology has been previously validated to detect lipid-rich plaque.[6,15] The studies included in this meta-analysis evaluate the effectiveness of NIRS as a tool to identify plaques and/or patients likely to experience future adverse events. It is hypothesized that detecting at-risk patients and prospectively treating vulnerable plaques could prevent future coronary events.

The predictive ability of NIRS has evolved from identification of vulnerable patients based on global lipid burden to identification of individual vulnerable plaques with the potential for secondary intervention. The earliest studies explored the prognostic value of identifying vulnerable patients based on findings of lipid-rich plaques without addressing the potential for plaque-level prognostic identification. However, these studies were relatively small and used different LCBI thresholds. Oemrawsingh and colleagues with a sample size of 203 patients was the first to identify the long-term prognostic value of NIRS as assessed in nonculprit vessels using an LCBI threshold of 43.0, representing the median.[8] The study reported a 1-year cumulative incidence of MACCE to be 16.7% in patients with an LCBI of 43 or greater versus 4.0% in those with an LCBI less than the threshold.

Schuurman and colleagues expanded on the findings of Oemrawsingh and colleagues, increasing the sample size to 275 by adding the IBIS-3-NIRS cohort to the original ATHEROREMO-NIRS cohort and increasing follow-up from 1-year to 4-year. The authors reported a statistically significant and independent continuous relationship between higher $maxLCBI_{4mm}$ values and a higher risk of MACE in a nontarget vessel using hazard ratios (HR). Each additional 100 units of $maxLCBI_{4mm}$ value was associated with a 19% increase in MACE (HR 1.19, 95% CI 1.07–1.32). This is similar to the findings from later studies such as Waksman and colleagues, which reported that there is an 18% increase in risk at the patient level for each 100-unit increase in $maxLCBI_{4mm}$ (HR 1.18, 95% CI 1.05–1.32) using a much larger sample size of 1271.

Waksman and colleagues further determined that NIRS can predict adverse outcomes at the individual plaque level by testing the association between $maxLCBI_{4mm}$ in a Ware segment, as defined in the study protocol, and occurrence of MACE within that same segment during the 24-month follow-up period. Waksman and colleagues showed each additional 100 units of $maxLCBI_{4mm}$

value at the plaque level was associated with a 45% increase in MACE (unadjusted HR 1.45, 95% CI 1.3–1.60). Erlinge and colleagues similarly corroborated this relationship with a 4-year Kaplan-Meier estimated rate of events that showed an increase in nonculprit lesion-related MACE according to baseline $maxLCBI_{4mm}$ in increments of 100. Erlinge and colleagues showed a 3.7% increased site-specific risk of MACE during a 4-year period from index presentation in patients with $maxLCBI_{4mm}$ between 400 and 500, a 5.7% increase in patients with $maxLCBI_{4mm}$ between 500 and 600, and a 10.4% increased risk in patients with $maxLCBI_{4mm}$ more than 600. The ability to prospectively identify risk of particular lipid-rich plaques makes for more robust risk prediction. An example patient case emphasizing the role of NIRS in risk prediction, modified from Waksman and colleagues, is described in **Fig. 1**. Further research may explore opportunities for intervention and treatment at the plaque-level to prevent future coronary events.

Lipid core burden index as a marker for therapy efficacy and response to therapy

NIRS has also demonstrated an ability to assess plaque modification by new pharmacologic therapies. In the PACMAN-AMI randomized clinical trial recently published by Räber and colleagues,[16] NIRS-derived $maxLCBI_{4mm}$ was used to show the superiority of alirocumab in reducing lipid core burden when given in addition to high-intensity statin versus high-intensity statin therapy alone. Mean change in $maxLCBI_{4mm}$ was −79.42 with alirocumab plus rosuvastatin and −37.60 with rosuvastatin alone after 52 weeks of therapy in patients with acute myocardial infarction (difference, −41.24, $P = .006$).[16] Particularly when used in conjunction with other imaging modalities such as IVUS and optical coherence tomography, NIRS allowed for valuable plaque level characterization that can be used in future studies to help evaluate the efficacy of novel treatments that may minimize complications at follow-up. As options for secondary prevention become more robust and efficacious, NIRS will have increasing importance as a strategy for both identifying high-risk patients and quantifying their response to treatment.

Lipid core burden index best cutoff associated with cardiovascular events

There have been different values defining elevated LCBI. Oemrawsingh and colleagues defined values above that of the median (LCBI > 43 in their study) as an elevated LCBI, which is relatively similar to the definition used by Danek and colleagues (LCBI $\geq$ 77). Madder and colleagues, Karlsson and colleagues, and Waksman and colleagues define elevated LCBI as a maxLCBI$_{4mm}$ greater than 400 with Schuurman and colleagues choosing a similar value of any LCBI at or above the fourth quartile (maxLCBI$_{4mm}$ $\geq$ 360). Erlinge and colleagues used the upper quartile maxLCBI$_{4mm}$ of 324.7 as the prespecified definition of lipid-rich plaque. Erlinge and colleagues furthermore explored a different definition to define vulnerable plaques as any plaque with maxLCBI$_{4mm}$ in the highest quartile plus plaque burden greater than 70% or small luminal area (defined as $\leq$ 4 mm^2). We recommend to always use the LCBI value as a marker of continuum risk and maxLCBI$_{4mm}$ greater than 400 to categorize patients/plaques as a high risk.

Limitations

There are several limitations that must be acknowledged: First, reliability and validity of the WebPlotDigitizer program has been questioned in prior studies at an aggregate level.[17] However, results in a 2016 study indicated high levels of intercoder reliability and validity.[18] To minimize this limitation, we relied on reported numbers for odds ratio calculations whenever possible. Second, the primary outcomes for each study include a range of LCBI value thresholds to determine the OR. We conducted the secondary analysis including studies with maxLCBI$_{4mm}$ thresholds around 400 to optimize the comparison. Although the NIRS binary cutoff of 400 maxLCBI$_{4mm}$ was confirmed as a reasonable predictor for subsequent events at the patient and plaque level in Waksman and colleagues, a definitive optimal threshold has yet to be determined. Third, the longest length of follow-up was a median of 5.3 years, with the majority of the identified studies with less than 4 years of follow-up. Many of the studies might have missed important LCBI-related adverse events due to short follow-up. More research is needed to determine the incidence of adverse events over time. Finally, we recognize that there exists a moderate level of heterogeneity between studies, as delineated with the I^2 statistical (58.7%).

SUMMARY

NIRS-derived LCBI is an effective measurement for identifying vulnerable patients and plaques at risk of future MACE/MACCE. Patients with an elevated LCBI have 2.93 times higher odds of enduring a future adverse event. The precision of the pooled OR provides a more precise estimate

that can be used in future studies. A maxLCBI$_{4mm}$ of 400 or greater seems to be a useful threshold for classifying at-risk plaques.

CLINICS CARE POINTS

- NIRS can identify particular patients at risk for future MACE/MACCE and provide an opportunity for risk stratification.
- NIRS-derived maxLCBI$_{4mm}$ > 400 can locate high-risk lipid-rich plaques and predict potential areas of future complication.
- NIRS has demonstrated an ability to assess plaque modification by new pharmacologic therapies and quantify patient responsiveness to treatment.

DISCLOSURE

H M. Garcia-Garcia reports the following Institutional grant support: Biotronik, Boston Scientific, Medtronic, Abbott, Neovasc, Shockwave, Phillips and Corflow. R Waksman: Advisory Board: Amgen, Boston Scientific, Cardioset, Cardiovascular Systems Inc., Medtronic, Philips, Pi-Cardia Ltd.; Consultant: Amgen, Biotronik, Boston Scientific, Cardioset, Cardiovascular Systems Inc., Medtronic, Philips, Pi-Cardia Ltd.; Grant Support: AstraZeneca, United Kingdom; Biotronik, Germany; Boston Scientific, United States; Chiesi, Italy; Speakers Bureau: AstraZeneca, Chiesi, Italy; Investor: MedAlliance. P Shah and S Sum are employees of InfraRedx, A Nipro Company. Other authors do not have conflicts of interest.

ACKNOWLEDGMENTS

Thank you to all co-authors for their expertise and assistance throughout each aspect of this analysis and for their help in drafting and editing the manuscript.

REFERENCES

1. Virani SS, Alonso A, Benjamin EJ, et al. Heart disease and stroke statistics—2020 update: a report from the american heart association. Circulation 2020;141(9):e139–596.
2. Finn AV, Nakano M, Narula J, et al. Concept of Vulnerable/Unstable Plaque. Arterioscler Thromb Vasc Biol 2010;30(7):1282–92.

3. Muller JE, Abela GS, Nesto RW, et al. Triggers, acute risk factors and vulnerable plaques: the lexicon of a new frontier. J Am Coll Cardiol 1994;23(3):809–13.

4. Virmani R, Kolodgie FD, Burke AP, et al. Lessons from sudden coronary death. Arterioscler Thromb Vasc Biol 2000;20(5):1262–75.

5. Wilkinson SE, Madder RD. Intracoronary near-infrared spectroscopy—role and clinical applications. Cardiovasc Diagn Ther 2020;10(5):1508–16.

6. Gardner CM, Tan H, Hull EL, et al. Detection of lipid core coronary plaques in autopsy specimens with a novel catheter-based near-infrared spectroscopy system. JACC: Cardiovasc Imaging 2008;1(5):638–48.

7. Moher D, Liberati A, Tetzlaff J, et al. Preferred reporting items for systematic reviews and meta-analyses: The PRISMA statement. Int J Surg 2010;8(5):336–41.

8. Oemrawsingh RM, Cheng JM, García-García HM, et al. Near-infrared spectroscopy predicts cardiovascular outcome in patients with coronary artery disease. J Am Coll Cardiol 2014;64(23):2510–8.

9. Madder RD, Husaini M, Davis AT, et al. Large lipid-rich coronary plaques detected by near-infrared spectroscopy at non-stented sites in the target artery identify patients likely to experience future major adverse cardiovascular events. Eur Heart J - Cardiovasc Imaging 2016;17(4):393–9.

10. Danek BA, Karatasakis A, Karacsonyi J, et al. Long-term follow-up after near-infrared spectroscopy coronary imaging: Insights from the lipid cORe plaque association with CLinical events (ORACLE-NIRS) registry. Cardiovasc Revascularization Med 2017;18(3):177–81.

11. Schuurman AS, Vroegindewey M, Kardys I, et al. Near-infrared spectroscopy-derived lipid core burden index predicts adverse cardiovascular outcome in patients with coronary artery disease during long-term follow-up. Eur Heart J 2018;39(4):295–302.

12. Karlsson S, Anesäter E, Fransson K, et al. Intracoronary near-infrared spectroscopy and the risk of future cardiovascular events. Open Heart 2019;6(1):e000917.

13. Waksman R, Mario CD, Torguson R, et al. Identification of patients and plaques vulnerable to future coronary events with near-infrared spectroscopy intravascular ultrasound imaging: a prospective, cohort study. Lancet 2019;394(10209):1629–37.

14. Erlinge D, Maehara A, Ben-Yehuda O, et al. Identification of vulnerable plaques and patients by intracoronary near-infrared spectroscopy and ultrasound (PROSPECT II): a prospective natural history study. Lancet 2021;397(10278):985–95.

15. Waxman S, Dixon SR, L'Allier P, et al. In vivo validation of a catheter-based near-infrared spectroscopy system for detection of lipid core coronary plaques: initial results of the spectacl study. JACC: Cardiovasc Imaging 2009;2(7):858–68.

16. Räber L, Ueki Y, Otsuka T, et al. Effect of alirocumab added to high-intensity statin therapy on coronary atherosclerosis in patients with acute myocardial infarction: the PACMAN-AMI randomized clinical trial. JAMA 2022. https://doi.org/10.1001/jama.2022.5218. Published online April 3.

17. Moeyaert M, Maggin D, Verkuilen J. Reliability, validity, and usability of data extraction programs for single-case research designs. Behav Modification 2016;40(6):874–900.

18. Drevon D, Fursa SR, Malcolm AL. Intercoder Reliability and validity of webplotdigitizer in extracting graphed data. Behav Modif 2017;41(2):323–39.

19. Stone GW, Maehara A, Lansky AJ, et al. A prospective natural-history study of coronary atherosclerosis. N Engl J Med 2011;364(3):226–35.

Moving?

Make sure your subscription moves with you!

To notify us of your new address, find your **Clinics Account Number** (located on your mailing label above your name), and contact customer service at:

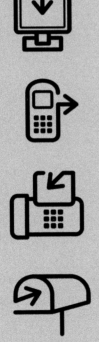

Email: journalscustomerservice-usa@elsevier.com

800-654-2452 (subscribers in the U.S. & Canada)
314-447-8871 (subscribers outside of the U.S. & Canada)

Fax number: 314-447-8029

Elsevier Health Sciences Division
Subscription Customer Service
3251 Riverport Lane
Maryland Heights, MO 63043

ELSEVIER

9780443183287